Airway Management in Emergency Medicine

Edited by Theodoros Aslanidis and Carlos Darcy Alves Bersot

Published in London, United Kingdom

Airway Management in Emergency Medicine
http://dx.doi.org/10.5772/intechopen.110971
Edited by Theodoros Aslanidis and Carlos Darcy Alves Bersot

Contributors
Theodoros Aslanidis, Vinicius Barros, Carlos Darcy A. Bersot, Gaurav Dhir, Mayank Dhir, Garima Jain, Nigar Kangarli, Asım Esen, Hiroaki Kume, Natsumi Watanabe, Yasuhito Suzuki, Erick Dunkley-Pinnock, Jorge Francisco Piña Rubio, María Elena Buenrostro Espinosa, Ricardo Serrano Tamayo, Jesus Cuevas Garcia, Ana Valentina Plascencia Gutiérrez, José David Durán Morales, Larry Chavira Calderon, Omolola Fagbohun

First published in London, United Kingdom, 2023 by IntechOpen
IntechOpen is the global imprint of INTECHOPEN LIMITED, registered in England and Wales, registration number: 11086078, 5 Princes Gate Court, London, SW7 2QJ, United Kingdom

British Library Cataloguing-in-Publication Data
A catalogue record for this book is available from the British Library

Additional hard and PDF copies can be obtained from orders@intechopen.com

Airway Management in Emergency Medicine
Edited by Theodoros Aslanidis and Carlos Darcy Alves Bersot
p. cm.
Print ISBN 978-1-83769-365-8
Online ISBN 978-1-83769-364-1
eBook (PDF) ISBN 978-1-83769-366-5

Meet the editors

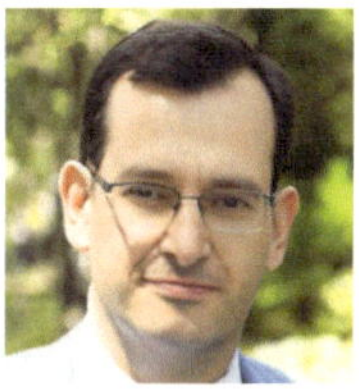

Theodoros Aslanidis received his MD from Plovdiv Medical University, Bulgaria, and his Ph.D. from Aristotle University in Greece. After serving as a medical doctor in the Hellenic Armed Forces and as a rural physician at Outhealth Centre, Iraklia and Serres General Hospital, Greece, he completed specialist anesthesiology training at Ippokrateio General Hospital, Greece; critical care sub-specialty training at AHEPA University Hospital, Greece; and a prehospital emergency medicine postgraduate program at the Hellenic National Centre for Emergency Care, Greece. He served as an EMS physician and emergency communication center medic before moving to his current post as consultant-researcher in the Intensive Care Unit at St. Paul General Hospital, Greece. He is also head of postgraduate studies at the College of Offshore and Remote Medicine, Malta.

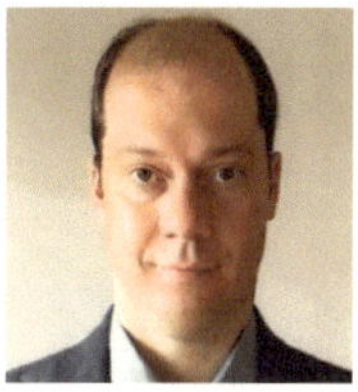

Carlos Darcy A. Bersot received his MD from the Faculty of Medicine of Campos (FMC), Brazil. He completed a residency in anesthesiology at the Hospital Federal da Lagoa, Brazil, where he is the head of the Medical Residency Program in Anesthesiology (CET/SBA). He is also an anesthesiologist at the Hospital for the Heart in Brazil. He obtained a specialty degree in anesthesiology from the Brazilian Society of Anesthesiology. He is an active member of the Brazilian Society of Anesthesiology (SBA) and the Society of Anesthesiology of the State of Rio de Janeiro (SAERJ). Dr. Bersot is a former Professor of Pain Sciences at the Faculty of Medicine, University of Valençia, Spain, and a former Professor of Pharmacology and Physiology at FMC. His main areas of expertise include neuroanesthesia, acute pain, and pharmacology. He is also a professor of point-of-care ultrasound at Artmed, Brazil.

Contents

Preface

Airway management is a critical component of emergency medicine, as it is essential to maintain oxygenation and prevent complications related to respiratory distress or failure. The dynamic character of an emergency and the lack of time for proper clinical evaluation and obtaining a complete medical history create unique challenges, even for the most experienced professionals. In addition, emergencies in limited-resource (regarding staff and equipment) environments further complicate the situation. And though many airway talks start at intubation, immediate intubation is rarely the first step in resuscitation. Proper assessment and basic airway maneuvers are also essential. Judicious utilization of pre- and apneic oxygenation is evenly important as is the choice of medications to facilitate intubation in this at-risk population.

The interest in airway management was further boosted by the COVID-19 pandemic and has continued to advance at a fast pace. Advances in video laryngoscopy, flexible intubation scopes, jet ventilation, and non-invasive ventilation measures such as high-flow nasal cannula apnoeic oxygenation and ventilation and nasal continuous positive airway pressure masks, have now reached every clinical specialty. Handheld point-of-care ultrasound facilitates rapid screening for difficult laryngoscopy, identification of the cricothyroid membrane for potential cricothyroidotomy, and assessment of increased aspiration risk, as well as confirmation of proper endotracheal tube positioning.

New concepts in the physiology of difficult airway, simulation training, as well as checklists and guidelines to identify patients with high-risk features (such as severe metabolic acidosis, shock and hypotension, obstructive lung disease, pulmonary hypertension, right ventricle failure, pulmonary embolism, and severe hypoxemia) and enhance patient safety, are now evolving.

This book provides comprehensive information on airway management in emergency situations, serving as a valuable guide for those involved in the management of similar cases.

Theodoros Aslanidis
Intensive Care Unit and Anesthesia Department,
"Agios Pavlos" General Hospital,
Thessaloniki, Greece

Carlos Darcy Alves Bersot
Anesthesia Department,
Hospital for the Heart,
São Paulo, Brazil

Chapter 1

Introductory Chapter: Pharmacology of Airway Management in Emergency Medicine

Theodoros Aslanidis, Vinicius Barros and Carlos Darcy A. Bersot

1. Introduction

Definite airway management in the majority of emergency cases means tracheal intubation. Yet, both laryngoscopy and intubation can provoke a series of physiological reflex responses due to posterior pharynx's afferent receptors (innervated by IX and X cerebral nerve). Central nervous system (CNS), cardiovascular system, and respiratory system responses to these stimuli vary in intensity; thus, it may potentially negatively affect patients' outcome.

Anesthesia is used to attenuate those responds and ease the procedure. A combination of different drugs and dosage regimens is used. Knowledge of efficacy, toxicity, therapeutic ratio, and special consideration of those drugs is essential in order to achieve optimal conditions in any given case [1].

2. Hypnosis

2.1 General considerations

An ideal induction anesthetic induction agent should be acting rapidly, yet smoothly without or with minimal respiratory and cardiovascular depression, and act protectively for brain circulation. Recovery should be rapid, with minimal or zero adverse effects and absence of any pain on injection.

Despite the tremendous progress in pharmacology development, we are still far from such a drug. Thus, the advantages and the limitation of the available drugs, in combination with the status of the patient, will determine the final choice [2].

2.1.1 Etomidate

Since its introduction in clinical practice in 1970, etomidate remains a valuable choice for emergency airway management due to its fast onset of action and minimal cardiovascular effects. It is mainly used in cases of hemodynamically fragile patients.

Its main drawbacks are nausea and prolonged suppression of adrenocortical steroid synthesis. Like propofol, etomidate interacts with GABA A receptors in a stereoselective way. Of all intravenous anesthetics used clinically, etomidate shows the greatest selectivity for GABA A receptors and has the fewest number of ionic interactions.

After intravenous injection, etomidate is tightly bound to plasma proteins such as albumin; plasmatic levels of cortisol, cortisone, and aldosterone are reduced, while those of 11-deoxycorticosterone, 11-deoxycortisol, and 17-hydroxyprogesterone are increased. Free drug is highly lipophilic, rapidly penetrating the blood-brain barrier; peak brain levels are reached 2 minutes after injection. Etomidate undergoes a hepatic metabolism (ester hydrolysis) to an inactive metabolite.

Etomidate central nervous system's effects are alike to those of propofol and barbiturates. During unconsciousness transmission (induction), loss of cortical inhibition may provoke myoclonus (that can be confused with generalized tonic-clonic seizures). Etomidate has anticonvulsant activity in several experimental models, yet smaller than propofol and thiopental. Despite its favorable hemodynamic profile, it should be noted that patients with elevated sympathetic tone, such as those suffering from shock, intoxication, or drug withdrawal, may experience an abrupt drop in blood pressure, even when the drug is used only to induce anesthesia [3, 4].

2.1.2 Thiopental

Thiopental is a thiobarbiturate that facilitates the GABA (an inhibitory neurotransmitter) transmission, thus causing reticular activating system depression. It is supplied as a sodium salt that requires preparation to solution before use. It is non-compatible with acidic solution (e.g., pancuronium or rocuronium—it will precipitate), and accidentally intra-arterial injection can cause less water solubility (forming crystals in the arterioles) leading to tissue necrosis.

Induction dose depends to volemic status (3 to 5 mg/kg in healthy euvolemic adults, 1 to 3 mg/kg in cases of hypovolemia). Onset is fast (30 seconds), and the duration of effect is 5 to 10 minutes. It is an ideal choice for patients with increased intracranial pressure (ICP), since it results a dose-dependent decrease in cerebral metabolic rate and cerebral blood flow. However, it has no analgesic effects, can induce bronchospasm (histamine release), has negative intropic effects, and may precipitate hypotention and venodilatation, thus making it a poor choice in sepsis. It has been shown to suppress white blood cell recruitment, activation, and activity *in vitro* and *in vivo*, but there are no reports of increased mortality in septic patients receiving a thiopental induction [5, 6].

2.1.3 Ketamine

Clinical effects observed after ketamine administration include elevations in blood pressure and muscle tone, eye opening (often accompanied by nystagmus), increased myocardial oxygen consumption, and minimal respiratory depression. Ketamine has no effect on laryngeal or pharyngeal reflexes, so the airways of the patient remain intact. It is also a potent bronchodilator and can be used to treat refractory bronchospasm.

The commercially available preparation is a racemic mixture. The S+ isomer has more potent anesthetic and analgesic properties, which reflects a fourfold higher affinity for N-methyl-D-aspartate (NMDA) receptor binding sites. Hepatic biotransformation of the S+ isomer is faster, contributing to a faster return of cognitive function.

Ketamine produces dose-dependent depression in the CNS, leading to the situation known as the "dissociative anesthetic state," which is characterized by inhibition of the thalamocortical system (deep analgesia and amnesia) and activation of the limbic system (delusional dreams).

Its use is recommended for induction of anesthesia in patients with asthma because of its ability to produce bronchodilation.

The renewed interest in ketamine is related to the use of lower doses (100–200 μg/kg) as an adjunct to anesthesia. Subanesthetic doses (0.1–0.5 mg/kg IV) produce analgesic effects. Ketamine's anesthetic (sedative) and opioid analgesic-sparing effects reduce ventilatory depression. Unlike barbiturates, which act on the reticular activating system in the brainstem, ketamine acts on receptors in the cortex and limbic system. The activity on NMDA receptors may be responsible for the analgesic action as well as the psychiatric effects (psychosis). Ketamine also has sympathomimetic activity, which results in tachycardia, hypertension, increased myocardial and cerebral oxygen consumption, cerebral blood flow, and intracranial and intraocular pressure.

Ketamine has a distribution phase about 45 minutes (highly perfused tissues>muscle>peripheral tissue>fat) and easily crosses the placenta. Ketamine's half-life is about 2 hours to 3 hours and has a primarily renal metabolism—kidneys (90%) and feces (5%), with 4% of an administered dose excreted unchanged in the urine.

When ketamine is administered intravenously, a sensation of dissociation is seen within 15 seconds, and anesthesia occurs within 30 seconds. Anesthesia lasts from 5 minutes to 10 minutes for intravenous administration. Ketamine's analgesic effects last from 20 minutes to 45 minutes. Anesthetic effects are eliminated by a combination of redistribution and hepatic biotransformation to a metabolite with only 30% of its activity.

Usage for anesthesia is 1 to 4.5 mg/kg of ketamine infused over approximately 60 seconds. On average, 2 mg/kg will produce 5 minutes to 10 minutes of surgical anesthesia. If a longer effect is desired, additional increments can be administered to maintain anesthesia without producing significant cumulative effects [7].

2.1.4 Propofol

Propofol (1,3-diisopropylphenol) is a non-barbiturate intravenous anesthetic that is chemically unrelated to other intravenous anesthetics. It is used to induce and maintain anesthesia and can be infused continuously until the end of the procedure. When administered into small-caliber peripheral veins, it causes pain in most patients.

Anesthesia with propofol has a rapid induction, similar to thiopental, but emergence from anesthesia is 10 times faster and is associated with minimal confusion postoperative. Only desflurane has a faster recovery time than propofol, but it is associated with nausea/vomiting.

The initial distribution half-life is 2 minutes to 4 minutes, and the elimination half-life is 1 hour to 3 hours. For a tricompartmental model, the initial distribution half-life is from 1 minute to 8 minutes and the slow distribution half-life is from 30 minutes to 70 minutes. The elimination half-life is dependent on the drug infusion time and ranges from 2 hours to 24 hours. Despite this long elimination half-life, the context-sensitive half-life of propofol is 40 minutes for infusions longer than 8 hours. Propofol is metabolized by the liver, forming inactive compounds, and is eliminated by the kidneys. Because it has a clearance greater than hepatic blood flow, it is believed to have other sites of metabolism in addition to the liver, possibly the lungs. The induction dose in adults is 1.5 to 2.5 mg/kg, and the plasma levels to reach unconsciousness are 2 to 6 μg/ml. The dose is higher in children and lower in the elderly and in patients with comorbidities. It will also be reduced with the administration of adjuvant drugs and/or opioids. The infusion rate for the maintenance of hypnosis ranges from 100 to 200 μg and for sedation from 25 to 75 μg/kg/min, at plasma concentrations of 1 to 1.5 μg/ml, usually when the plasma concentration drops by 50% of the initial one [8].

3. Analgesia

3.1 Opioids

Although it is not recommended as part of the classic rapid sequence induction technique, use of opioids will attenuate the cardiovascular responses to laryngoscopy and intubation. This may be particularly valuable if intracranial pressure is raised or the patient has a history of coronary artery disease. Usually, opioid administration decreases the dose of an induction agent.

In case of apnea due to respiratory depression and a "cannot intubate" situation, reversal with naloxone may be required.

Fentanyl is a potent (100 times more potent than morphine) synthetic opioid with a relatively fast onset (2–5 min), short duration of action (30–60 min after a single dose), and minimal cardiovascular effects (still, a chance of bradycardia exists). A usual dose of 2–3 μg/kg IV will usually reduce the rise in blood and intracranial pressure, triggered by laryngoscopy and intubation. Alfentanil (usual dose 10–20 μg/kg iv) reaches its peak action after just 90 seconds (duration: 5–10 minutes), which make it a good alternative to fentanyl. Finally, remifentanil is even more potent opioid that can be used either as alternative to fentanyl (doses 0.5–1 μg/kg) or even as alternative to rapid-onset paralytic agents (succinylcholine or rocuronium) in higher doses (3–4 μg/kg) for rapid sequence intubation. Morphine, on the other hand, may be used in addition to, or instead of midazolam, ketamine or etomidate in cases of ventilatory difficulty secondary to combativeness in already intubated patients; yet it is not considered a useful agent for emergency airway management.

4. Neuromuscular blocking drugs (NMBs)

4.1 Suxamethonium (or succinylcholine)

Suxamethonium (1.5–2 mg/kg) is the only depolarizing agent in use, with fast onset (starting at 15 seconds and complete block in 45–60 sec, short duration (4–6 minutes), and high potency. It still—after more than 50 years since its introduction into clinical practice—remains the drug of choice for neuromuscular blockade during rapid sequence intubation (RSI), though rocuronium is gaining more and more popularity. It is metabolized by plasma pseudocholinesterase ($T_{1/2}$—47 sec) to succinylmonocholine and choline. Its main drawbacks are the side effects it may provoke:

- Hyperkalemia that increase by up to 0.5 mmol/l even in normal subjects. This increase in potassium concentration may be greatly in patients with certain pathological conditions, particularly demyelinating conditions, desquamating skin conditions, major trauma, burns, and several other pathologies (muscle myopathies) where loss of muscle excitation secondary to denervation, immobilization, or inflammation leads to up-regulation of immature acetylcholine (Ach) receptors throughout the whole muscle membrane.

- Bradycardia, which is especially if large or repeated doses are given, children are most at risk. Thus, atropine should be ready for administration. Children do not need to be pretreated with atropine routinely but draw up the correct dose (0.02 mg kg^{-1}) and be ready to give it whenever a child is anesthetized.

- Muscle fasciculation that can increase intracranial, intraocular, and intragastric pressure. The effect could be attenuated when proper dose of induction drug is given concurrently.

- Muscle pain that likely to occur 12–24 hours after giving suxamethonium to fit young patients and those who mobilize quickly after anesthesia.

- Histamine release that may cause significant hypotension in some patients

- Prolonged neuromuscular block, which is in patients with low or abnormal pseudocholinesterase activity or in cases with repeated doses of suxamethonium, paralysis may be prolonged. The action of suxamethonium may also be prolonged in the presence of organophosphate poisoning or cocaine use, when neuromuscular blockade may last from 20 to 30 minutes.

4.2 Non-depolarizing muscle relaxants (ndNMB)

ndNMB agents have several properties that may affect airway function (**Table 1**) There are two major categories: steroidal (rocuronium, vecuronium and pancuronium) and benzylisoquinolinium (cisatracurium, atracurium, and mivacurium). Though there are a lot of available ndNMB, the vast majority of them is used only for cases with no airway emergency. Of note also is the fact that these agents pose various effects, with the diaphragm and the adductor muscles of the larynx being more resistant to paralysis than some of the muscles affecting upper airway patency. The most common side effect is histamine release, which clinically includes hemodynamic instability (tachycardia and hypotension), bronchospasm, and urticaria. Several drug interactions should also be in mind when using ndNMB: drug-like antibiotics (aminoglycosides, clindamycin, and tetracycline), antiarrhythmics (quinidine and calcium channel blockers), dantrolene, ketamine, local and inhaled anesthetics, and magnesium sulfate augment their action, while anticonvulsants (phenytoin, valproic acid, and carbamazepine), cholinesterase inhibitors (neostigmine and pyridostigmine) inhibit their potency.

Contraindications include cerebral palsy, burn injuries, hemiplegia, peripheral nerve injury, and severe chronic infections of botulism or tetani that induce resistance and conditions like advanced life support (ALS), autoimmune disorders, Guillain-Barre, Duchenne type muscular dystrophy, or myasthenia gravis which trigger hypersensitivity.

Muscle relaxants	Type	Typical induction dose (mg/kg)	Time to onset (minutes)	Duration to 25% recovery
Succinylcholine	Depolarizer	1–1.5	1–1.5	6–8
Rocuronium	Nondepolarizer	0.9–12	1–1.5	30–40
Vecuronium	Nondepolarizer	0.08–12	3–4	35–45
Cisatracurium	Nondepolarizer	0.1–0.15	5–7	30–45
Pancuronium	Nondepolarizer	0.08–0.12	2–4	60–120

[a] *Typical times to onset and recovery, and induction doses of common muscle relaxants are compared. Recovery time is defined as the time to regain 25% of baseline movement elicited by electrical stimulation.*

Table 1.
Commonly used non-depolarizing neuromuscular blockers [1].

The only nNMB that is gaining interest and popularity for airway emergencies is rocuronium and 1.0–1.2 mg kg^{-1} of rocuronium can be used for modified rapid sequence induction, and will enable intubation after 60 seconds, with duration of 45–60 min. Its use was further boosted with the introduction of suggamadex (see below). Yet, even then RSI is best performed by senior staff, and with an acceptance that timely progression to surgical airway may be required.

4.3 Sugammadex

Sugammadex is a steroidal nNMB binder, a cyclodextrin that works by binding NMB molecules in a 1:1 ratio and has designed to reverse steroidal ndNMBs, while the neostigmine/glycopyrrolate combination is still in use for the reversal of benzyliso-quinolinium ndNMB. The complex formed is excreted by kidneys.

Usual dosing in 4–8 mg/kg (causing reversal in about 3 min) yet immediate reversal of rocuronium after RSI requires a large dose of sugammadex (i.e., 16 mg/kg). In the obese patient, the dose should be based on actual body weight. If decision of reintubation is made then a 30-min waiting time after sugammadex reversal appeared to be the cutoff to decrease the onset time to less than 2 min if an RSI dose of 1.2 mg/kg for rocuronium is used. Otherwise, benzylisoquinolinium ndNMB or succinylcholine should be used.

Sugammadex is costly, and its side effects include hypersensitivity, effects on hemostasis (with an increased risk of bleeding in some patient groups), and bradycardia. Furthermore, the use of sugammadex for immediate reversal of rocuronium in children and adolescents has not been investigated.

5. Others

5.1 Esmolol

Esmolol is a short-acting cardioselective beta-1 receptor antagonist effective in reducing the adrenergic response to various perioperative stimuli, including laryngoscopy for tracheal intubation and tracheal extubation. Several studies have demonstrated the beneficial effects of esmolol on analgesia, but the mechanism has not yet been fully elucidated. One hypothesis is that under physiological conditions, nociceptors are not activated by sympathetic stimulation. With inflammation after surgery, catecholamines sensitize nociceptors and modulate neurogenic inflammatory responses, important in primary and secondary hyperalgesia. Beta-adrenergic antagonists are possible blockers of the excitatory effects of noradrenaline [9]. Beta-adrenergic antagonists can also modulate central adrenergic activity and calcium and potassium channels in the central nervous system, generating some types of central analgesia [10–12]. During laryngoscopy for orotracheal intubation, the beneficial effects are more restricted to the attenuation of undesirable hemodynamic effects.

Studies have shown that esmolol, when used in continuous infusion, is effective in reducing undesirable hemodynamic effects such as hypertension and tachycardia during laryngoscopy maneuvers for orotacheal intubation [13–15]. Esmolol was also associated with lower intraoperative opioid consumption [16, 17].

Esmolol can also be a safe drug to be used at the time of extubation, especially in patients sensitive to hemodynamic effects such as tachycardia and hypertension. Mendonça et al. in 2021 demonstrated that in patients undergoing surgery during the extubation maneuver, esmolol was effective in attenuating these effects by not delaying extubation [15].

In this context, esmolol can be a safe option, sparing opioids, to be used both in orotracheal intubation, intraoperatively and postoperatively for most patients, and its short half-life brings yet another advantage, as it increases safety even more of this medication.

6. Regional and topical anesthesia of the airway

Though there are a lot of regional and topical techniques that may in reality provide conditions for awake endotracheal intubation (application techniques such as the McKenzie technique that uses a 20-gauge cannula attached to oxygen bubble tubing *via* a three-way tap or a mucosal atomization device for spraying local anesthetic, and glossopharyngeal nerve or superior laryngeal nerve or recurrent laryngeal or translaryngeal block), they are time-consuming, thus limiting their use in emergency situations.

Author details

Theodoros Aslanidis[1]*, Vinicius Barros[2] and Carlos Darcy A. Bersot[2]

1 Intensive Care Unit/Anesthesiology Department, St. Paul General Hospital, Thessaloniki, Greece

2 Department of Anesthesiology, Hospital for the Heart, São Paulo, Brazil

*Address all correspondence to: thaslan@hotmail.com

References

[1] George RB, Hung OR. Chapter 4. Pharmacology of intubation. In: Hung O, Murphy MF, editors. Management of the Difficult and Failed Airway. 2nd ed. New York, United States: McGraw Hill; 2012

[2] Consilvio C, Kuschner WG, Lighthall GK. The pharmacology of airway management in critical care. Journal of Intensive Care Medicine. 2012;**27**(5):298-305. DOI: 10.1177/0885066611402154

[3] McCollum JS, Dundee JW. Comparison of induction characteristics of four intravenous anaesthetic agents. Anaesthesia. 1986;**41**:995-1000

[4] Choi SD, Spaulding BC, Gross JB, et al. Comparison of the ventilatory effects of etomidate and methohexital. Anesthesiology. 1985;**62**:442-447

[5] Sivilotti ML, Ducharme J. Randomized, double-blind study on sedatives and hemodynamics during rapid-sequence intubation in the emergency department: The SHRED study. Annals of Emergency Medicine. 1998;**31**(3):313-324

[6] White PF, Romero G. Nonopioid intravenous anesthesia. In: Barash P, Cullen B, Stoelting R, editors. Clinical Anesthesia. 9th ed. Philadelphia, United States: Wolters Klover; 2023

[7] Fackler JC, Arnold JH. Anesthetic Principles and Operating Room Anesthesia Regimens. In: Fuhman BP, Zimmerman J. Pediatric Critical Care. 3rd Ed. Philadelphia: Mosby Elsevier; 2006

[8] Sgrò S, Morini F, Bozza P, Piersigilli F, Bagolan P, Picardo S. Intravenous Propofol allows fast intubation in neonates and young infants undergoing major surgery. Frontiers in Pediatrics. 2019;**7**:321. DOI: 10.3389/fped.2019.00321

[9] Pertovaara A. The noradrenergic pain regulation system: A potential target for pain therapy. Euro J Pharmacol. 2013;**15**(716):2-7

[10] Hageluken A, Grunbaum L, Nurnberg B, Harmhammer R, Schunack W, Seifert R. Lipophilic beta-adrenoreceptor antagonists and local anesthetics are effective direct activators of G-proteins. Biochemical Pharmacology. 1994;**47**:1789-1795

[11] Chia YY, Chan MH, Ko NH, Liu K. Role of beta-blockade in anesthesia and postoperative pain management after hysterectomy. British Journal of Anesthesia. 2004;**93**:799-805

[12] Huang WJ, Moon YE, Cho SJ, Lee J. The effect of a continuous infusion of Loa-dose esmolol on the requirement for remifentanil during laparoscopic gynecologic surgery. Journal of Clinical Anesthesia. 2013;**25**:36-41

[13] Hamed JME, Ataalla WM. Esmolol infusion reduces blood loss and opiate consumption during fertility preserving myomectomy. Anesthesia, Essays and Researches. 2019;**13**(3):423-429. DOI: 10.4103/aer.AER_118_19

[14] Sharma S, Suthar OP, Tak ML, Thanvi A, Paliwal N, Karnawat R. Comparison of Esmolol and Dexmedetomidine for suppression of hemodynamic response to laryngoscopy and endotracheal intubation in adult patients undergoing elective general surgery: A prospective, randomized controlled double-blinded study.

Anesthesia, Essays and Researches. 2018;**12**(1):262-266. DOI: 10.4103/aer.AER_226_17

[15] Mendonça FT, Barreto Filho JH, Hungary MBCS, Magalhães TC. Efficacy of a single dose of esmolol to prevent extubation-related complications during emergence from anesthesia: A randomized, double-blind, placebo-controlled trial. Braz J Anesthesiol. 2021;**73**(4):426-433. DOI: 10.1016/j.bjane.2021.08.012

[16] Gelineau AM, King MR, Ladha KS, Burns SM, Houle T, Anderson TA. Intraoperative Esmolol as an adjunct for perioperative opioid and postoperative pain reduction: A systematic review, meta-analysis, and meta-regression. Anesthesia and Analgesia. 2018;**126**(3):1035-1049. DOI: 10.1213/ANE.0000000000002469

[17] Morais VBD, Sakata RK, Huang APS, Ferraro LHDC. Randomized, double-blind, placebo-controlled study of the analgesic effect of intraoperative esmolol for laparoscopic gastroplasty. Acta Cirúrgica Brasileira. 2020;**35**(4):e202000408. DOI: 10.1590/s0102-865020200040000008

Chapter 2

A Panoramic View of Airway Management in Emergency Medicine

Gaurav Dhir, Mayank Dhir and Garima Jain

Abstract

Airway management is a fundamental skill for emergency medical professionals like paramedics, EMTs, and emergency physicians. It involves quickly evaluating and addressing airway obstructions or breathing difficulties, often in high-stress, life-threatening situations. Proficiency requires a deep understanding of airway anatomy, physiology, and interventions, along with adaptability and rapid decision-making. This chapter summarizes evidence on key aspects, including assessing difficult airways, positioning, oxygenation, intubation methods, medications, devices, and rescue strategies, across various patient groups. Effective airway management is crucial for enhancing patient outcomes and reducing mortality in emergencies.

Keywords: airway management, difficult airway, airway devices, supra glottic airway devices, direct laryngoscopy, video assisted laryngoscopy, eFONA, airway pharmacology

1. Introduction

Emergency airway management is critical in emergency medicine, with securing the airway as the top priority for critically unstable patients. Around 0.5–1% of ED visitors require intubation due to conditions like respiratory failure, cardiac arrest, and altered mental state. ED intubation presents unique challenges, including vomiting, facial/neck injuries, cervical spine immobilization, and chest compressions. These factors impact intubation success, emphasizing the need for ED physicians to understand current evidence. Evidence underscores achieving first-pass intubation success, discouraging multiple attempts, which elevate risks like adverse events, higher failure rates, reduced chances of ROSC, and prolonged resuscitation times. Adequate preparation and assessing difficult airways are crucial for successful intubation. This chapter explores first-pass success, airway management algorithms, and systematic rescue intubation strategies.

2. Applied anatomy

The pharynx, connecting nasal and oral cavities to the larynx and esophagus, comprises the nasopharynx, oropharynx, and laryngopharynx. Obesity and a receding mandible can alter the airway, with excess fat affecting pharyngeal muscles and obstructing it. Enlarged tongues in obese individuals can pose challenges in mask ventilation. Negative intrathoracic pressure in obesity can further constrict the pharyngeal airway, worsening mask ventilation. The larynx, consisting of membranes, cartilage, and muscles, connects the respiratory and digestive tracts, safeguarding the airway and enabling speech. It includes nine cartilages, such as paired (arytenoid, corniculate, cuneiform) and unpaired (thyroid, cricoid, epiglottis). The thyroid cartilage forms the Adam's apple, while the cricoid cartilage lies below it, both crucial for airway procedures and nerve blocks.

The cricothyroid membrane, located between the cricoid and thyroid cartilages in the neck, plays a significant role in anatomy and clinical practice. In emergencies with compromised upper airways, cricothyroidotomy becomes essential, involving an incision in the cricothyroid membrane to establish a temporary airway, serving as a life-saving intervention when conventional methods fail [1–5].

The tracheobronchial tree, responsible for gas transport from the trachea to the lung's gas exchange units (acini), features a complex branching system. The trachea, extending from the C6 level to the carina, divides into the right and left main bronchi at the carina. The right main bronchus takes a more direct path and divides into smaller branches earlier, increasing the risk of inadvertent right endobronchial intubation during intubation.

3. Secured airway

A secured airway encompasses all necessary measures to establish and sustain an unobstructed air passage, ensure effective patient ventilation, and maintain oxygenation levels above 94%. This comprehensive approach encompasses the utilization of positioning techniques and a variety of airway adjunct tools, both basic and advanced, to ensure optimal patient respiratory function and safety (**Figure 1**) [6].

3.1 Signs of blocked airway

Recognizing signs of a blocked airway is crucial for prompt intervention. These indicators include mild tachypnea, visible retractions in the suprasternal and supraclavicular areas, nasal flaring, alterations in voice such as hoarseness or a barking cough, the presence of inspiratory stridor, limited chest expansion, reduced air entry during auscultation, and the emergence of cyanosis, excessive drooling, or persistent

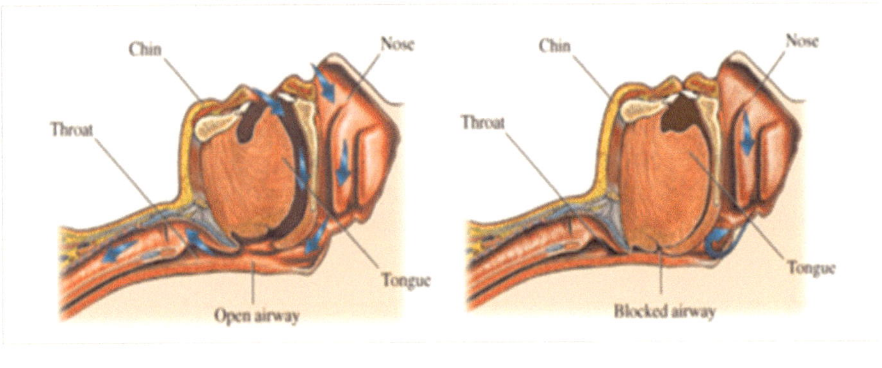

Figure 1.
Open airway vs. blocked airway.

coughing. Identifying these symptoms allows for timely action to ensure adequate airflow and prevent potentially life-threatening respiratory complications.

3.2 Techniques of securing an airway

Securing an airway aims to establish and maintain an open path for air to enter and exit the lungs. The approach varies based on severity and patient condition. Endotracheal intubation, inserting a tube into the trachea via mouth or nose, is a common method ensuring a protected airway with ventilation control. When intubation is not possible, supraglottic airway devices or bag-mask ventilation serve as viable alternatives.

3.3 Basic airway maneuvers

Basic airway maneuvers play a critical role in managing airway obstructions. The primary causes of blockage often involve the tongue or epiglottis displacement. Techniques like head tilt-chin lift and jaw thrust help establish a clear airway by repositioning the tongue and soft tissues. It's essential to exercise caution when employing these maneuvers, especially if there's a suspicion of cervical spine injury, as they can exacerbate the condition. For head tilt-chin lift, gently tilt the head back by pressing down on the forehead while lifting the chin with the index and middle fingers. For jaw thrust, place your palms on the temples, with fingers under the jaw, and lift the mandible upward to elevate the tongue. In children, a modified approach is used, with head tilt-chin lift without overextension and jaw thrust with just the index finger on the lower jaw. Combining head tilt, jaw thrust, and mouth opening creates the Triple airway maneuver, further enhancing airway clearance and maintenance.

3.4 Non definitive and definitive airway

The Non-Definitive airway category encompasses airway management techniques and devices that are positioned above the laryngeal inlet. Examples include oropharyngeal airways, nasopharyngeal airways, and supraglottic airway devices like the Combitube, Laryngeal tube, and LMA (Laryngeal Mask Airway). These tools and techniques are employed to establish and maintain a patent airway, particularly when definitive airway management may not be immediately necessary or feasible [7].

The Definitive airway category encompasses techniques and devices positioned below the laryngeal inlet, ensuring a secure and reliable airway. Examples include endotracheal tubes (both nasotracheal and orotracheal), tracheostomy, and cricothyroidotomy. These methods are utilized when there is a critical need to establish a secure and long-term airway, such as in cases of prolonged ventilation, surgical access, or severe upper airway obstruction.

3.5 Non definitive airway

3.5.1 Oropharyngeal airway (OPA, Guedel's airway)

An oropharyngeal airway is an airway adjunct used to maintain or open the airway by stopping the tongue from covering the epiglottis. It can potentially bypass airway obstruction caused by any of the oral structures like tonsillar hypertrophy, or falling back of tongue into the posterior pharynx in the supine position. The tip of the OPA should lie just above the epiglottis at correct insertion depth.

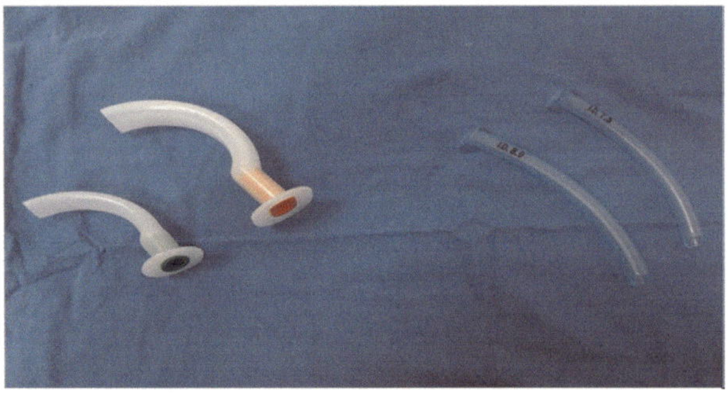

Figure 2.
Oropharyngeal and nasopharyngeal airway.

Its primary indication lies in its use for unconscious patients who struggle to maintain an open airway despite attempted airway maneuvers. However, it's essential to note that there are contraindications to its usage, namely conscious patients or those with an intact gag reflex, for whom alternative airway management methods should be considered. While the oropharyngeal airway can be lifesaving, it's not without potential complications. If improperly sized, it may induce gagging, retching, or even laryngospasm. Moreover, using an OPA that is too small might exacerbate airway obstruction by pushing the tongue backward (**Figure 2**).

3.5.2 Nasopharyngeal airway (NPA)

Nasopharyngeal airways are plastic hollow or soft rubber tubes can be utilized to aid difficult bag valve mask ventilation. They are passed through the nose to the posterior pharynx. The direction of insertion should be straight back towards the occiput and along the nasal floor rather than cephalad, with the concave side facing down to allow it to pass into the posterior pharynx behind the tongue.

Nasopharyngeal airways are typically indicated for awake or semi-conscious patients who possess an intact gag reflex, individuals with limited mouth opening due to conditions like trismus or angioedema, and those with fragile dentition. However, there are clear contraindications that should be adhered to, including patients with basilar skull fractures, facial trauma, or disruption of the midface, nasopharynx, or roof of the mouth, as well as individuals with coagulopathies or those taking anticoagulants due to an elevated risk of bleeding. Large nasal polyps and a history of recent nasal surgery also stand as contraindications. As with any medical procedure, potential complications must be considered, which can encompass trauma to nasal mucosa or adenoids leading to epistaxis, as well as the risk of gastric distension and vomiting if an excessively long device is employed (**Figures 3** and **4**).

3.5.3 Supraglottic airway devices (also known as extraglottic or periglottic devices)

Supraglottic Airway Devices (SGD) are devices that ventilate patients by delivering oxygen above the level of the vocal cords. The chief advantage of the supraglottic airway devices in emergency airway management include ease of placement by both experienced and inexperienced personal and hands free airway. As a rescue airway in difficult airway, failed intubation and cannot ventilate cannot intubate (CVCI) situations. There are many ways to classify SGD and one of them is according to there sealing mechanism (functional classification) [8].

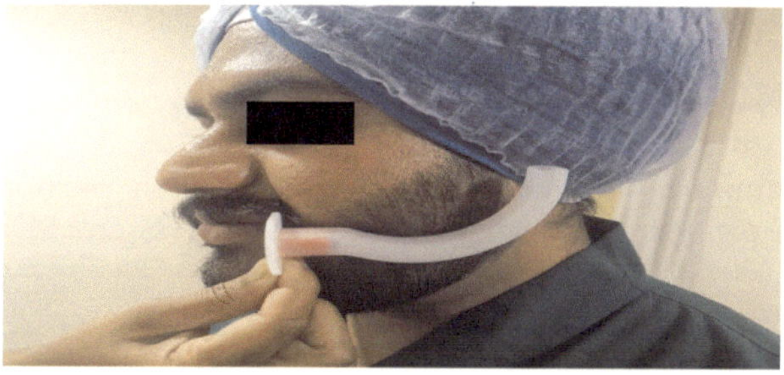

Figure 3.
Correct size assessment: The flange of the airway should be approximated,externally, to where it is abutting the lips, and the tip should be able to reach the angle of the mandible/ tragus of the ear.

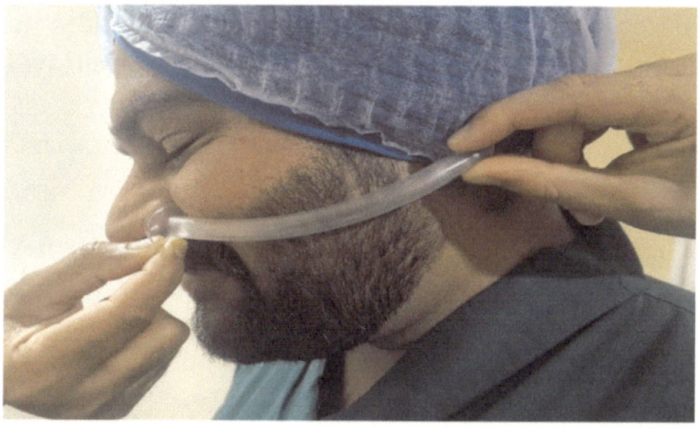

Figure 4.
Correct size assessment can be done placing flange at nasal opening and orienting the device towards the angle of the mandible/tragus of the ear.

- **Cuffed perilaryngeal sealer**
    - Non-directional non esophageal Sealers- cLMA, Flexible LMA, LMA unique.
    - Directional Non-esophageal sealing- Fastrach LMA, ALMA.
    - Directional esophageal sealing- Proseal LMA, Supreme LMA.
- **Cuffed pharyngeal sealer**
    - Without esophageal sealing: COPA, PAX.
    - With esophageal sealing: Combitube, Laryngeal tube, LTS.
- **Cuff less preshaped sealer**
    - With esophageal sealing- Baska mask, i-gel.
    - Without esophageal sealing- SLIPA, AirQ-ILA.

This chapter will provide a brief description of the top five supraglottic devices commonly utilized in emergency departments: cLMA, LMA Fastrach, Air Q ILA, i-gel, and Esophageal Combitube.

3.5.3.1 LMA classic (cLMA)

The Classic Laryngeal Mask Airway (LMA) is a widely used medical device designed to establish a secure and effective airway during various surgical and medical procedures. It features an inflatable cuff that, when properly positioned, seals the laryngeal inlet, allowing for ventilation and oxygenation (**Figure 5**).

3.5.3.2 Insertion technique

Inserting the Classic LMA is a relatively straightforward procedure. Hold the device like a pen, positioning your index finger at the junction of the cuff and airway tube. Gently press the cuff's tip upward against the hard palate while maintaining visual guidance, ensuring it flattens against the palate. With your index finger, press the cuff backward towards the occiput, advancing the device into the hypopharynx. Continue the insertion until your finger reaches its fullest extent within the oral cavity, taking care to stop before encountering resistance.

3.5.3.3 LMA Fastrach

LMA Fastrach has proven to be an effective airway device both within and outside the emergency room. Effective ventilation is rapidly and successfully established in nearly all cases and blind intubation is possible in majority of cases if optimal technique is used. Adjunct such as fiber optic bronchoscope or light wand may be used occasionally (**Figure 6**).

3.5.3.4 Insertion technique

Gently insert the LMA Fastrach into the patient's mouth, following the natural curvature of the tongue. Avoid using excessive force, as this can cause trauma. As you insert the LMA Fastrach, advance it gently until resistance is felt. Then, slightly rotate it 90 degrees, which helps align the tip with the laryngeal inlet.

Chandy's maneuver: It involves a series of precise steps for blind intubation via LMA Fastrach. The first step, the 1st Chandy's maneuver, focuses on optimizing ventilation by directing the airway aperture towards the glottis, ensuring efficient airflow. Following this, the 2nd Chandy's maneuver involves lifting the device vertically for proper positioning. Next, a well-lubricated wire-reinforced tube, with the black line oriented towards the patient's nose, is passed through. The cuff is then inflated, and placement is confirmed by monitoring end-tidal CO_2 levels. To secure the endotracheal tube (ETT),

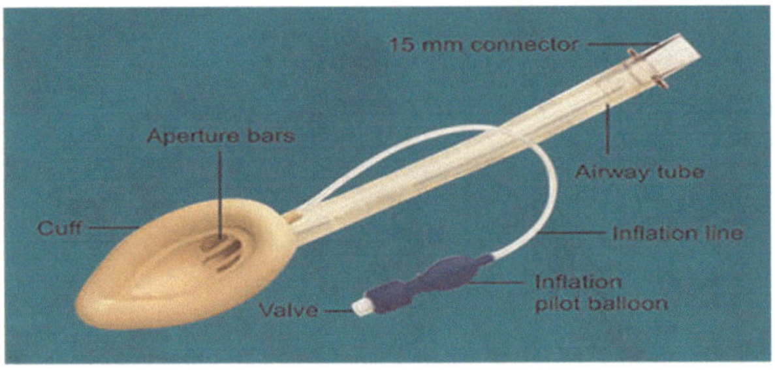

Figure 5.
Classic LMA.

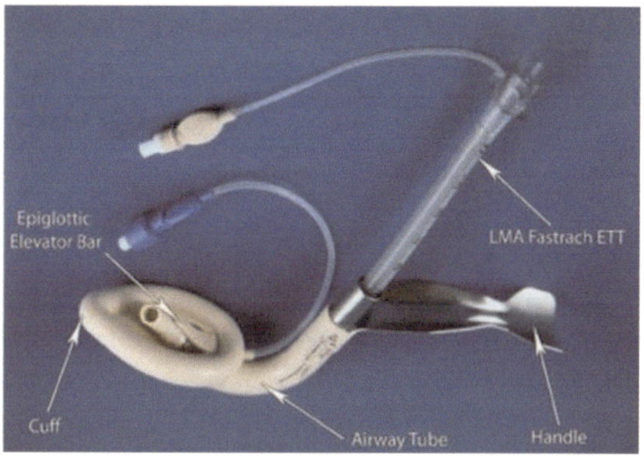

Figure 6.
LMA Fastrach.

the obturator rod is used for stabilization. Finally, the Laryngeal Mask Airway (LMA) is deflated and carefully removed, completing the Chandy's maneuver, a meticulous process critical for successful airway management [9].

3.5.3.5 Air-Q intubating laryngeal airway

Air -Q ILA was introduced by Daniel Cook in 2005 as an aid for airway maintenance and as a conduit for endotracheal intubation during general anesthesia. In case of intubation failure AirQ ILA can be used as a definitive airway (**Figure** 7).

3.5.3.6 Insertion technique

Hold the Air-Q LMA like a pen, with your index finger at the junction of the cuff and airway tube. Gently insert the device into the patient's mouth, following the natural curvature of the tongue. Aim to place the device so that the cuff sits within the hypopharynx and the airway tube is aligned with the laryngeal inlet.

To intubate via Air-Q LMA, first, disconnect the connector, and then introduce an appropriately sized and well-lubricated endotracheal tube (ETT). This can be accomplished either through blind insertion or with the assistance of a fiberoptic bronchoscope

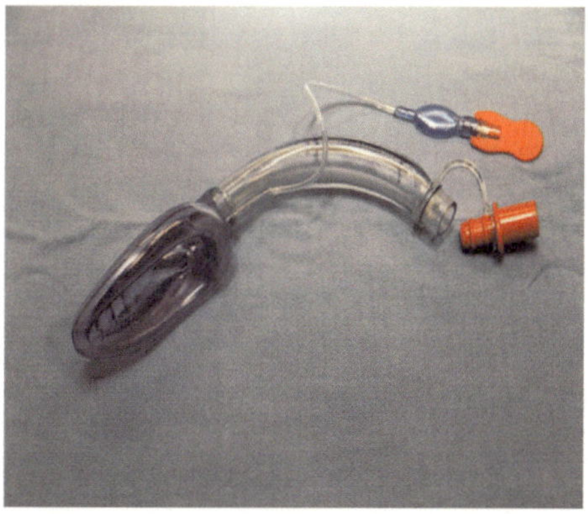

Figure 7.
Air-Q ILA.

for precision. Once the ETT is securely in place, deflate the cuff of the Air-Q ILA, use the AIR-Q removal stylet to stabilize the ETT, and subsequently remove the AIR-Q ILA from the patient's airway. This sequence of steps ensures a smooth and controlled transition from the Air-Q ILA to the ETT while maintaining optimal airway management.

3.5.3.7 I gel

I gel is made from a medical grade thermoelastic polymer, it has been designed to create a non inflatable anatomical seal of the pharyngeal, laryngeal and perilaryngeal structures while avoiding compression trauma. It houses separate airway tubing and gastric channels. The gastric channel allows suction of gastric contents and passage of a gastric tube (**Figure 8**).

3.5.3.8 Insertion technique

Grasp the device along the integral bite block and introduce into the mouth towards the hard palate, gliding downwards and backwards along the palate until a definite resistance is felt.

3.5.3.9 Esophageal combitube

The combitube is now primarily used for emergency airway management in prehospital settings as well as in CVCI situations in the hospital setting. It differs from other supraglottic airway devices in being designed for blind placement in either the trachea or the esophagus. It is a double lumen tube with2 cuffs, with one lumen opening beyond the distal cuff, while the other ending between the 2 cuffs with only side openings. The proximal high volume (blue) pharyngeal cuff is inflated with 85-100 ml air while the distal (white) with12-15 ml. The proximal cuff occludes the hypopharynx while the distal occludes either the trachea or the esophagus (**Figure 9**).

3.5.3.10 Insertion technique

To ensure proper placement of the airway device, maintain the patient's head in a neutral position and gently insert the device into the mouth in a downward curving motion until the teeth or gum line align with the two black lines on the device. Following insertion, inflate both cuffs with the appropriate volumes. Verify

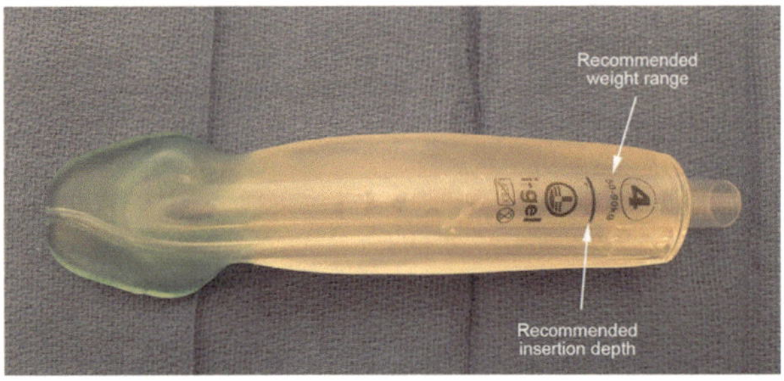

Figure 8.
I-gel.

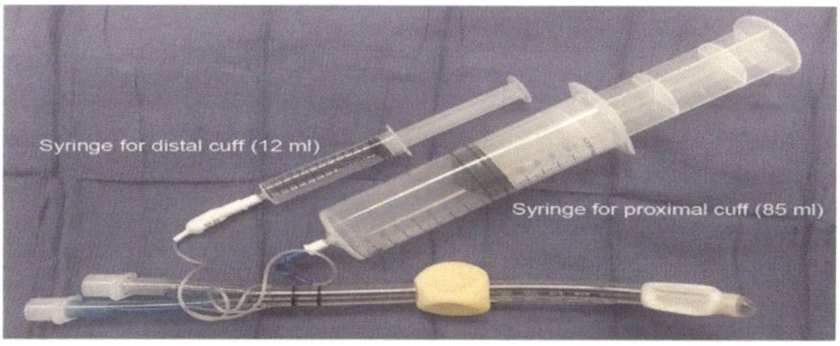

Figure 9.
Esophageal Combitube.

ventilation using the blue lumen: in the correct esophageal position, no gurgling should be audible over the epigastrium, and breath sounds should be detectable in the lung fields. If the distal cuff is in the trachea, gurgling will be heard in the epigastrium, and chest auscultation will reveal an absence of breath sounds. If neither breath sounds nor gurgling is present, it indicates that the tube has been inserted too far into the esophagus. To confirm tracheal placement, check ventilation using the clear lumen: if the distal cuff is in the trachea, there should be no gurgling, and breath sounds should be audible in the lung fields. Continue ventilation through the appropriate lumen that allows for effective ventilation.

3.6 Definitive airway

Endotracheal intubation is a common method used to create a definitive airway. This technique involves the insertion of a tube into the trachea, either through the mouth or nose, to maintain an open air passage. Intubation allows for precise control of ventilation and protects the airway from potential obstructions. Other approach to achieve a definitive airway in emergency care include cricothyroidotomy, which involves making an emergency incision in the cricothyroid membrane to access the airway. In the following discussion, we will explore various aids and techniques that assist in achieving a successful intubation procedure.

3.6.1 Endotracheal intubation aids

Endotracheal intubation may be achieved by any of the following airway aids depending upon the situation, device availability and operator expertise

- Direct laryngoscopy and intubation
- Bougie/Stylet guided intubation
- Lightwand guided intubation
- Video laryngoscopy and intubation
- Fibreoptic bronchscope guided intubation
- Supraglotic airway guided intubation

3.6.2 Direct laryngoscopy

Laryngoscope blades are essential instruments used during endotracheal intubation procedures to visualize the larynx and facilitate the insertion of an endotracheal tube. There are several different types of laryngoscope blades, each with its own unique design and purpose. The most commonly used blades include,

- **Macintosh**: This curved blade is the traditional choice for laryngoscopy. It has a smooth, curved tip that allows the blade to lift the epiglottis and visualize the vocal cords.

- **Miller**: The Miller blade is straight and has a flatter profile compared to the Macintosh blade. It is often used in pediatric cases or in patients with limited neck mobility. The straight design helps lift the epiglottis directly, providing a clear view of the vocal cords [10].

- **Mac Coy**: Hinged tip helps in elevating the epiglottis leading to an increased increased view of the larynx, useful in patients with anterior larynx

- **Polio Blade**: Very useful in intubating patients with breast hypertrophy, obese patients, patients with short neck and with restricted neck mobility [11].

- **Video Laryngoscope**: Unlike traditional direct laryngoscopy, which relies on a direct line of sight, video laryngoscopes incorporate a small camera at the tip of the blade or handle. This camera captures a real-time video image of the airway, which is displayed on a screen, allowing direct visualization of the larynx and guide the insertion of the endotracheal tube (**Figures 10–12**).

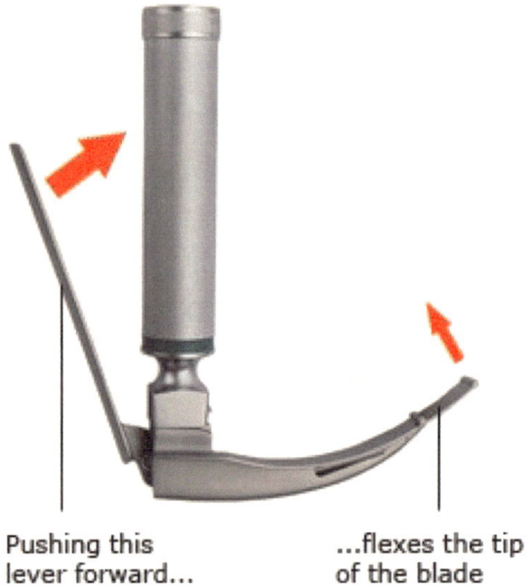

Figure 10.
McCoy laryngoscope blade.

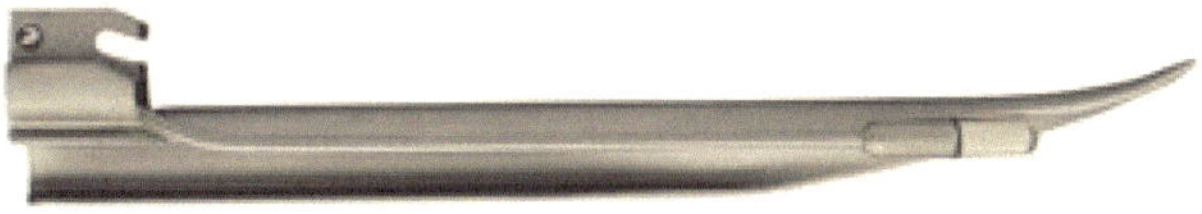

Figure 11.
Miller laryngoscope blade.

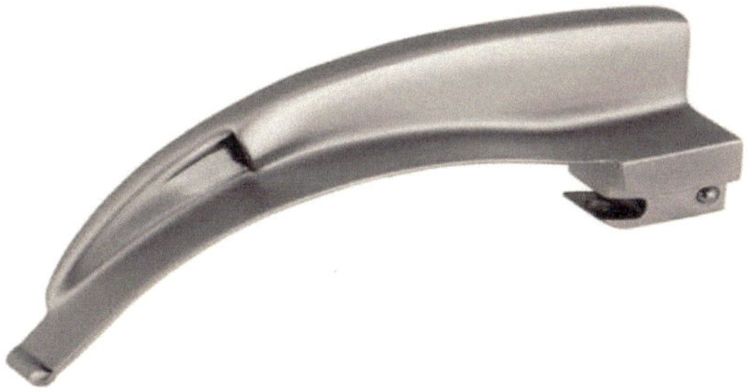

Figure 12.
Macintosh laryngoscope blade.

3.6.3 Bougie and stylets

When the larynx is only partially visualized or hidden behind the epiglottis at direct laryngoscopy, and may be difficult to reach with the normal curvature of an endotracheal tube, intubation may then be accomplished by either (**Figures 13–16**).

- Altering the curvature of the ETT using a malleable plastic coated metal Stylet.
- Inserting a long thin Gum Elastic Bougie (GEB) and using this as a guide over which the tube may be railroaded into the trachea.

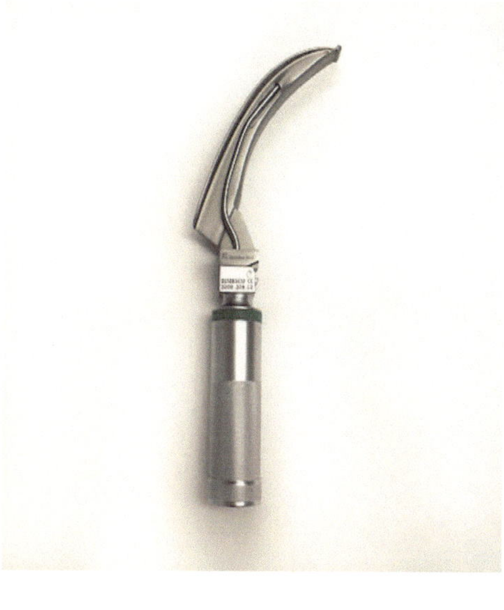

Figure 13.
Polio Macintosh laryngoscope.

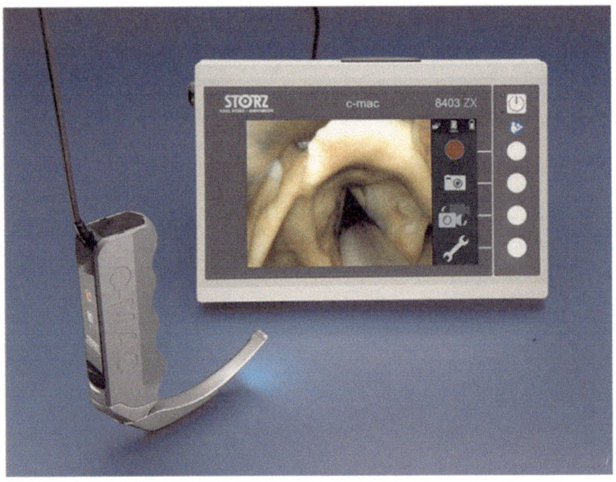

Figure 14.
Video laryngoscope.

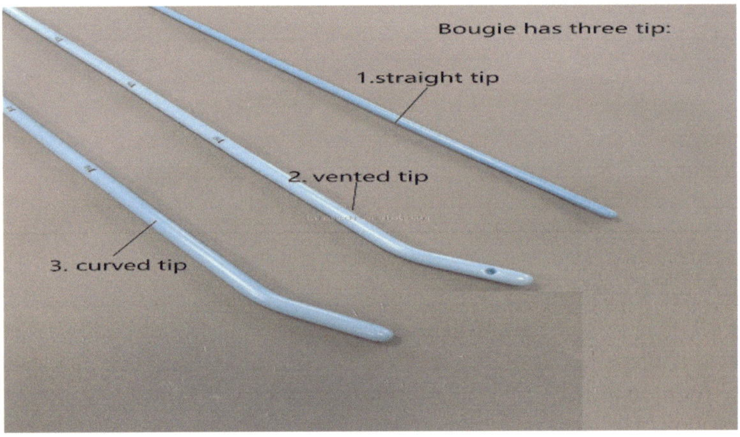

Figure 15.
Intubating stylets of different sizes(Fr).

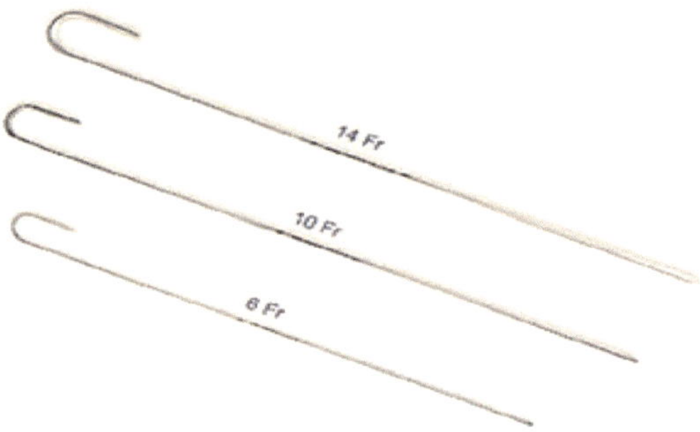

Figure 16.
Gum elastic Bougie.

3.6.4 Lightwand

It is an illuminated stylet which is introduced into the ETT and the tip of the tube is directed into the trachea guided by transillumination of neck tissues.

Lighwand tracheal intubation is a suitable method for difficult intubation in patients with

- Restricted cervical spine movement
- Limited mouth opening
- Orofacial distortion
- Unexpected failed intubation

3.6.5 Fibreoptic bronchoscope guided intubation

Fiberoptic bronchoscopes are currently used to facilitate endotracheal intubation via either the nasal or oral route (**Figure 17**). In clinical scenarios in which tracheal intubation is deemed necessary and mask or supraglottic ventilation (e.g., via a laryngeal mask airway [LMA]) is unlikely to be successful or poses an aspiration risk, awake FOI is a standard approach. FOI remains the accepted standard in emergency airway management of a patient with an anticipated difficult airway. FOI is ideally suited in such patients because intubation can be performed prior to the induction of anesthesia with its attendant risks of inadequate ventilation and oxygenation, loss of upper airway patency, and failed intubation. This FOI technique also safeguards against the risk of the cannot intubate/cannot ventilate scenario (**Figure 18**) [12].

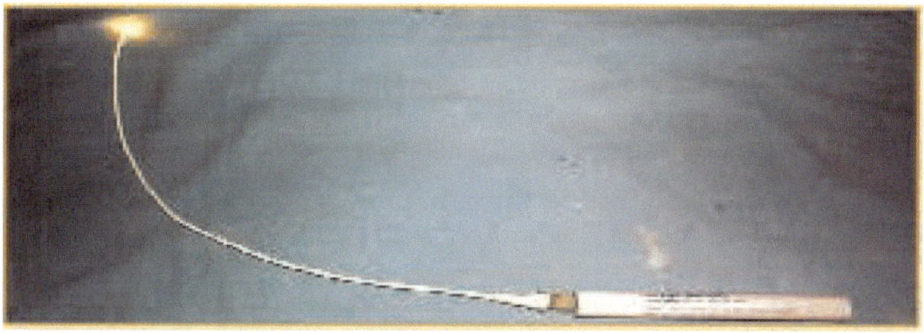

Figure 17.
Lightwand.

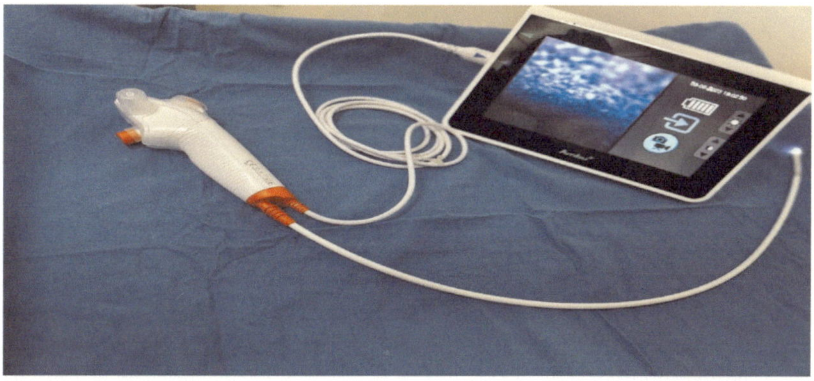

Figure 18.
AMBU fiberoptic bronchoscope.

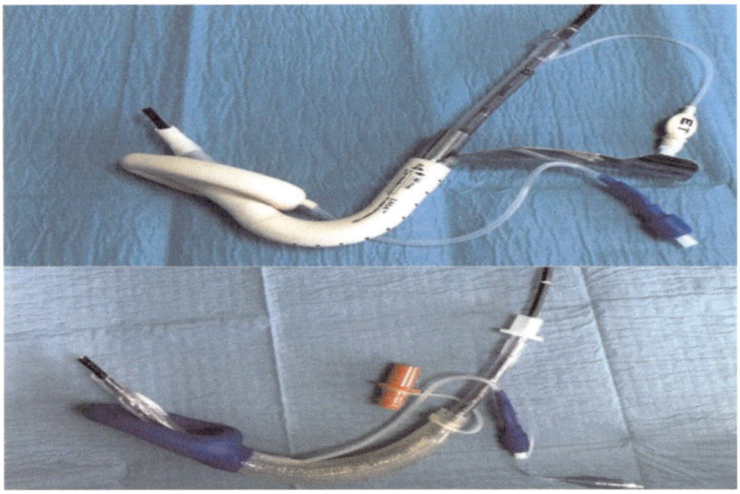

Figure 19.
Intubation via LMA Fastrach(above) and AIR-Q LMA(below).

3.6.6 Supraglotic airway guided intubation

Supraglottic device aids intubation by establishing initial airway, then guides endotracheal tube. Ensures clear, protected ventilation passage. Useful in challenging laryngoscopy or difficult airways. Effective alternative for secure intubation in clinical scenarios (**Figure 19**) [13].

4. Indications for securing a definitive airway

Broadly, the indications for intubating a patient can be remembered and categorized by the mnemonic:

A. **Airway Compromise.** When other methods fail to maintain a clear airway, and there is a risk of airway obstruction or compromise. This may occur in cases of inhalation injury, facial fractures, or retropharyngeal haematoma. In cases of dynamic airway early intubation is the key point.

- Bullets: Neck trauma
- Bites: Anaphylaxis/Angioedema
- Burns: Thermal and caustic airway injury

B. **Breathing.** Inadequate Oxygenation or Ventilation: When the patient cannot achieve sufficient oxygenation through the use of a face mask and supplemental oxygen, or when there is apnea (cessation of breathing).

C. **Circulation.** Inadequate Circulation & Cerebral Hypoperfusion: To enhance tissue oxygen delivery by relieving the respiratory muscles. This is necessary when the patient is experiencing decreased mental status or combativeness due to reduced blood flow to the brain.

D. **Disability.** CNS Depression due to any reason like Head Injury, CNS catastrophes, etc. In cases where the patient has a Glasgow Coma Scale (GCS) score of 8 or less, indicating severe obtundation resulting from a head injury. This may also be necessary in situations of prolonged seizure activity, neuromuscular weakness, or to protect the airway from aspiration of blood or vomit.

E. **Expected course.** Anticipated deterioration in the patient's condition or transfer to radiology or another institution.

F. **Feral.** The need for immediate aggressive sedation to protect the patient/others.

5. Algorithms for airway management

Algorithms are there for managing the airway, they provide a basic pathway for different intubation scenarios. It is vital that all clinicians who attempt intubation be familiar with the equipment and techniques necessary for successful intubation (**Figures 20–22**).

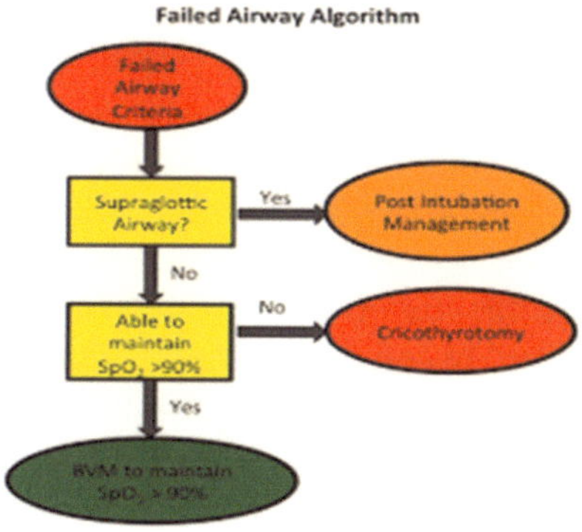

Figure 20.
Failed airway algorithm.

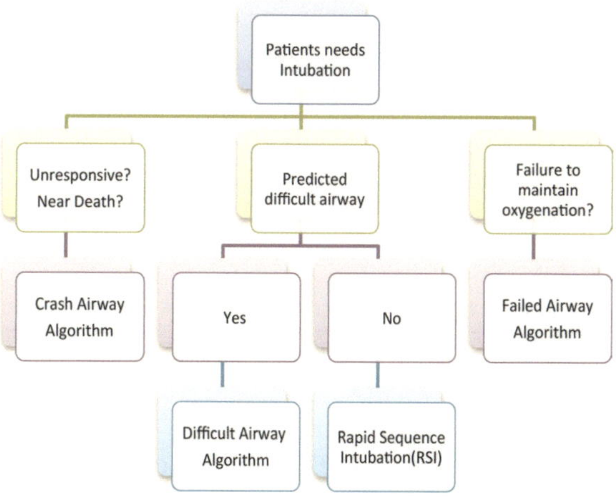

Figure 21.
Basic pathway for different intubation scenarios.

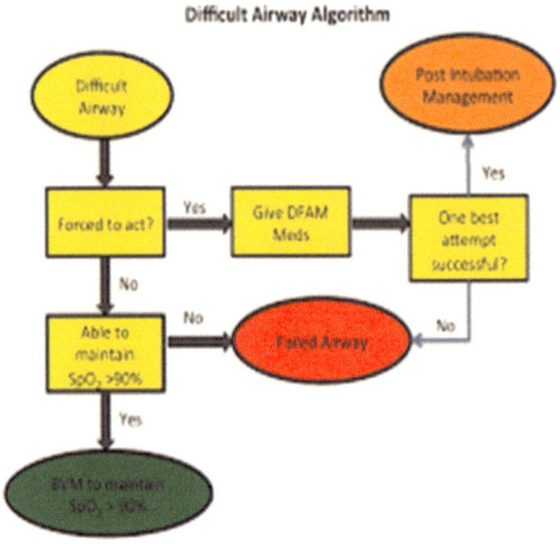

Figure 22.
Difficult airway algorithm.

6. Rapid sequence intubation (RSI)

It is a technique of intubation where in the airway is secured quickly and safely while reducing the risk of aspiration. Rapid sequence intubation is the standard method in emergency airway management for patients without an anticipated difficult airway.

Classic Rapid Sequence Intubation (RSI) and Modified RSI are two approaches to securing the airway in emergency and critical care settings. In Classic RSI, a standardized drug sequence, typically involving a rapid-acting induction agent followed by succinylcholine, is used, often with the application of cricoid pressure. In contrast, Modified RSI is more flexible, allowing for variations in drug choices and their order based on the patient's condition and provider's judgment. It may include positive pressure ventilation before paralysis and may avoid cricoid pressure. The choice of paralytic agents can also differ, with non-depolarizing agents like rocuronium sometimes preferred. Modified RSI emphasizes individualized care and adaptability to the clinical context, while Classic RSI follows a more standardized protocol. The approach chosen depends on factors such as patient condition, clinician expertise, and local protocols.

6.1 Conduct of RSI

- Preparation
- Pre oxygenation
- Intravenous anesthesia induction
- Cricoid pressure/Sellick's maneuver (The esophagus is blocked in an extended neck by pressing the cricoid cartilage against the 5th cervical vertebra.

Apply 10–40 N (1–4 kg) pressure using thumb and index finger post-induction until intubation and cuff inflation. Contraindicated in patients suspected with cervical spine injury or laryngeal injury [14]).

- Laryngoscopy followed by intubation after the requisite time has elapsed or by observing fasciculations.

- Confirmation of correct tube placement by 4 phase capnography waveform for at least 5 breaths or auscultation of chest.

7. Delayed sequence intubation

Delayed Sequence Intubation (DSI) is a specialized airway management technique used in emergency medicine and critical care when traditional rapid sequence intubation (RSI) may not be immediately feasible or safe. DSI is employed to optimize the patient's oxygenation and ventilation before initiating RSI. It is typically employed in cases where the patient presents with severe respiratory distress, hypoxemia, or impending respiratory failure. These situations may include agitated or combative patients who cannot cooperate with the standard RSI procedure (**Figure 23**) [15].

8. Crash intubation

Crash airway refers to patients in cardiopulmonary arrest, deep coma or near death who cannot maintain their ventilation and oxygenation (**Figures 24–26**).

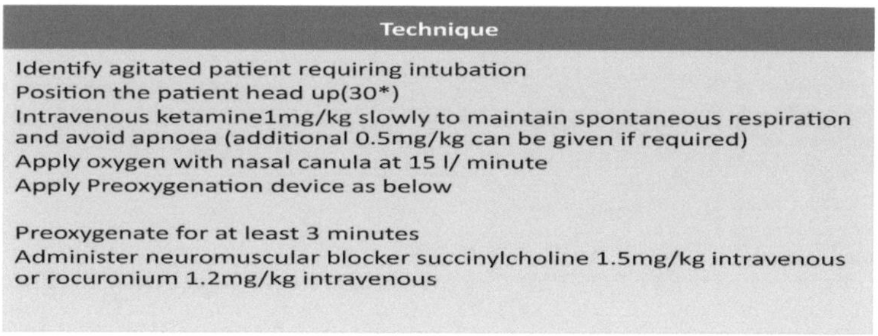

Figure 23.
Delayed sequence intubation technique.

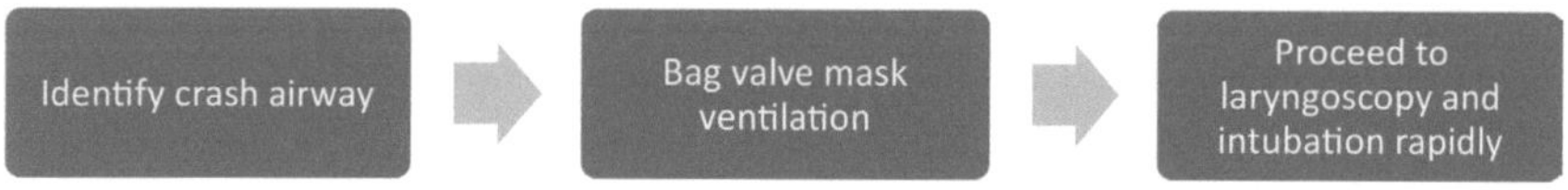

Figure 24.
Crash intubation.

9. Pre intubation preparation

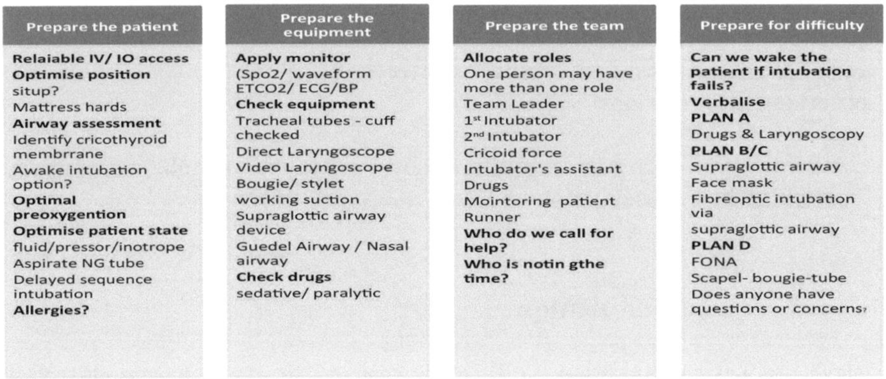

Figure 25.
Preintubation prepration.

10. Predictors of a difficult airway

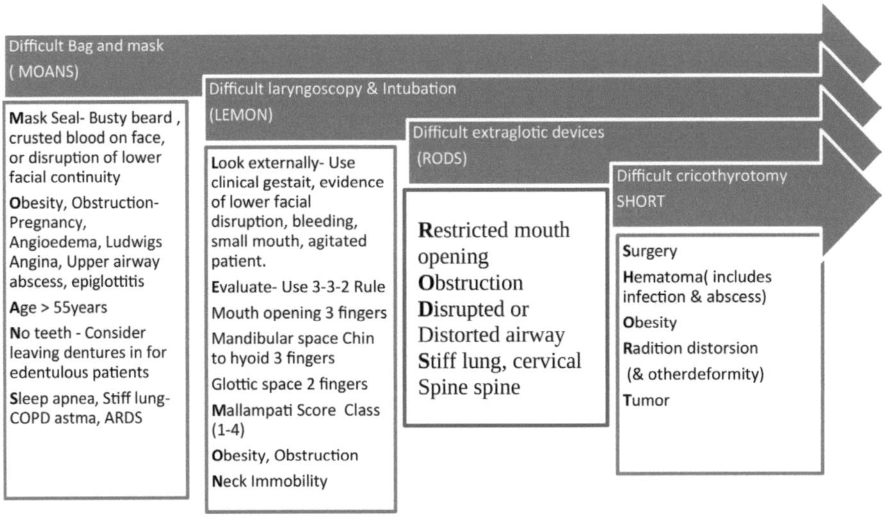

Figure 26.
Predictors of a difficult airway.

11. Preintubation positioning

Before performing intubation, it is crucial to position your patient correctly. Unless your patient is undergoing chest compressions due to cardiac arrest, optimizing the positioning prior to intubation is essential. Improved positioning enhances your view and increases the likelihood of a successful intubation on the first attempt, minimizing the risk of complications. Elevate the patient to the operator's xiphoid level for optimal positioning. While ventilation and intubation are typically done with the patient lying flat on their back, aligning the external ear with the sternal notch may enhance the visibility of the glottis. Avoid using padding under the shoulders or neck as this position is not ideal for facilitating emergency intubation. The goal of laryngoscopy is to align the oral, pharyngeal, and laryngeal axes to achieve a clear and unobstructed view of the glottis, enabling the passage of the endotracheal tube (ETT) between the vocal cords.

11.1 Scenario 1: Normal body position and the sniffing position

Positioning theory is centered on aligning three axes: the oral axis (OA), pharyngeal axis (PA), and laryngeal axis (LA). When a patient lies flat, their OA guides your line of sight to the oropharynx. In the sniffing position, achieved by using towels or blankets to flex the cervical spine and align the external auditory meatus with the sternal angle, these three axes come into alignment. This reduces the force needed to clear the glottis opening during intubation (**Figure** 27) [16].

11.2 Scenario 2: the overweight patient and the ramp

Overweight patients need special positioning attention, especially for the sniffing position due to excessive force for pharyngeal tissue displacement. Their heavier chest wall poses ventilation challenges and shortens safe apnea time. Elevating the torso with a ramp, using linens or pillows, helps slide chest wall tissues, improving preoxygenation and extending desaturation time. The ramped position, with the head at a 30-degree angle and the ear canal level with the sternum, benefits obese patients during intubation, as research shows advantages regardless of body mass index (BMI) (**Figure 28**) [17].

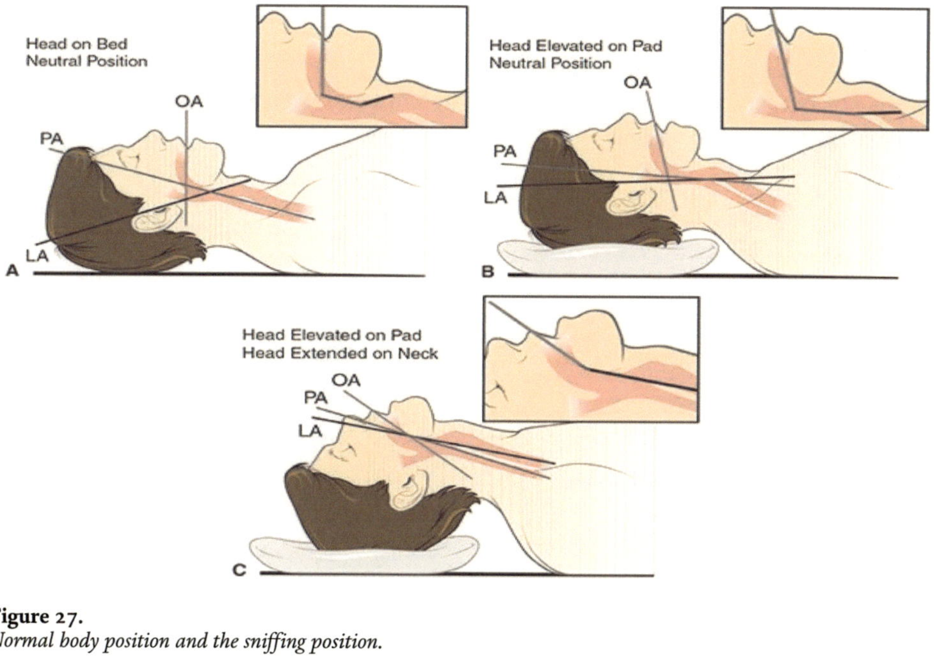

Figure 27.
Normal body position and the sniffing position.

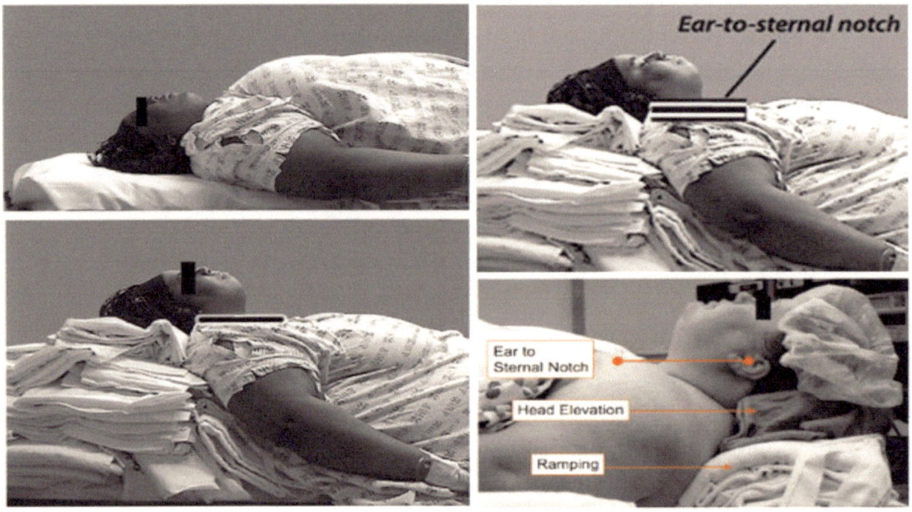

Figure 28.
The ramp position.

12. Pre intubation optimisation of oxygenation

When oxygen falls below 70%, it raises risks like dysrhythmias, decompensation, and cardiac arrest (**Table 1**). Pre-oxygenation removes alveolar nitrogen, creating an oxygen reserve, preventing hypoxia. In healthy patients, it extends safe apnea time to 8 minutes, but it's shorter for critically ill patients. Start preoxygenation before intubation, administering 100% oxygen for ≥3 mins at ≥15 L/min. Adjust the regulator to maximum "flush" for 90–97% oxygen at 40-60 L/min. Use tidal volume breathing with a proper seal. If >95% O2 is not achieved, consider bag-valve-mask ventilation, PEEP valves, or CPAP. Tilting the head 20–30 degrees upward enhances preoxygenation. For agitated patients, consider sedation or induction agents. During laryngoscopy, high-flow oxygen maintains airflow from the pharynx to the lungs [18].

	Device	% Fio_2 Obtained	Flow (L/min)
1	Nasal Cannula	24–40%	1–6
2	Face mask	35–60%	5–10
3	Oxymizer	24–45%	1–15
4	Venturi mask	24–50%	2–15
5	Non-rebreather mask	50–90%	10–15
6	High flow nasal cannula	30–100%	15–60
7	BIPAP	35–100%	
8	Endotracheal Intubation	35–100%	

Table 1.
Various oxygenation delivery devices.

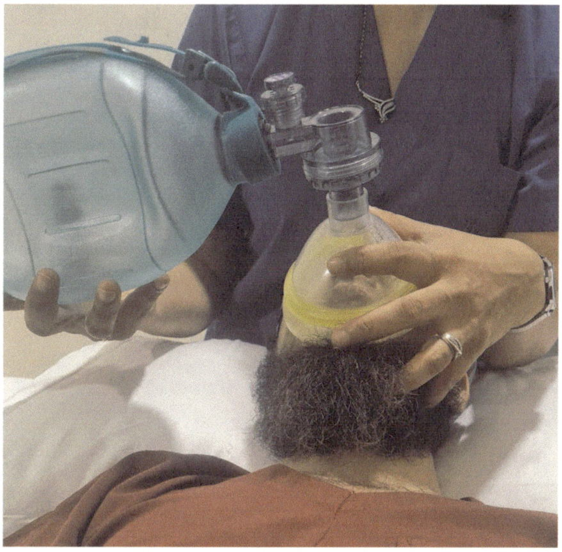

Figure 29.
Single rescuer bag mask ventilation (E-C).

12.1 Bag valve mask ventilation

Bag-valve mask ventilation is essential for airway management by various medical professionals. Techniques like denture retention, beard lubrication, and airway adjuncts aid in challenging situations. It delivers positive pressure ventilation to patients with inadequate breaths, excluding those with total airway obstruction or aspiration risk. Perform with the patient supine and the head in a sniffing position (except for cervical spine injury). Two techniques:

One-person: Seal the mask to the patient's face using the E-C method.

Two-person: One squeezes the bag, and the other maintains the mask seal, avoiding neck compression and ensuring pressure on bony points. Proper positioning matters; larger masks improve the seal, while smaller ones may leak. Complications can include gastric insufflation leading to vomiting and aspiration (**Figures 29** and **30**).

13. Vortex approach

The Vortex approach to airway management has been designed to assist decision making during airway crisis (**Figure 31**). It follows the principle that if the non-surgical methods (tracheal intubation, SAD, and facemask ventilation) for achieving alveolar oxygenation fail, there is diminishing time and options available before critical hypoxaemia occurs. If a best effort at any of these is unsuccessful, the 'CICO status' is initiated and preparation for eFONA starts, and failure of the best effort in all three should initiate eFONA [19].

14. Emergency front of neck access [eFONA]/surgical airway

About 3% of intubation attempts are challenging, necessitating consideration of a surgical airway when endotracheal intubation fails. In these emergencies, securing the

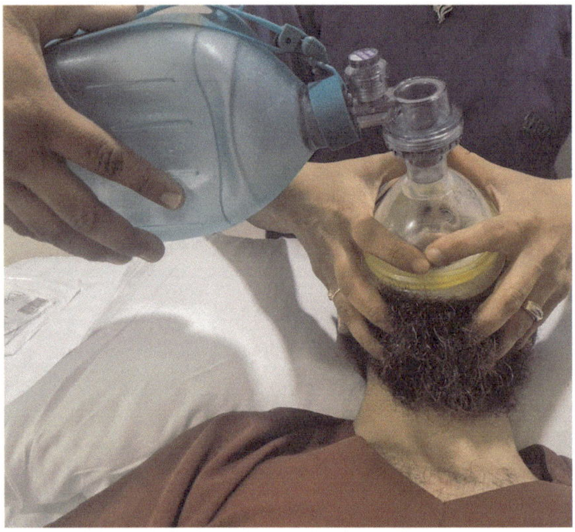

Figure 30.
Two rescuer bag mask ventilation.

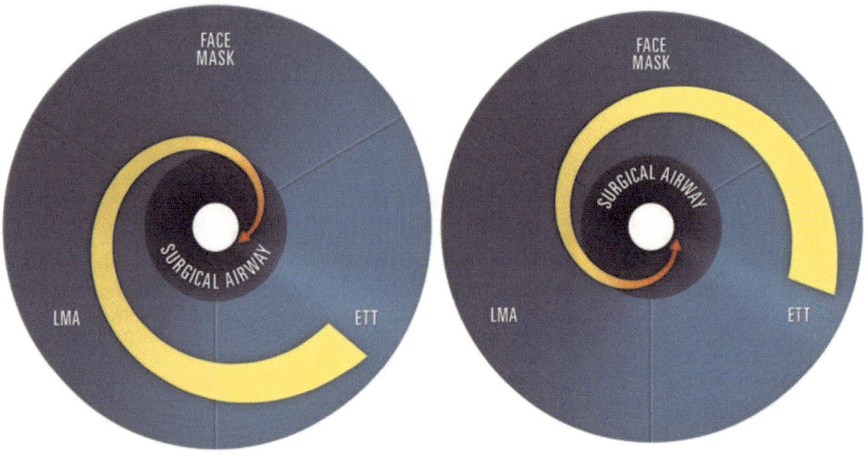

Figure 31.
Use of vortex during failed RSI.

airway is crucial for saving lives. Accessing the airway through the front of the neck typically involves cricothyrotomy (needle, scalpel-bougie, transtracheal catheter, or surgical) or tracheostomy (surgical or percutaneous), with an emphasis on the cricothyroid membrane. This approach is recommended and included in the difficult airway algorithm for situations where other airway management methods have failed, such as "can't intubate, can't oxygenate" (CICO) scenarios. It can also be performed electively before anesthesia induction in awake patients with upper airway obstruction, severe injuries, or high CICO risk (**Figure 32**) [19].

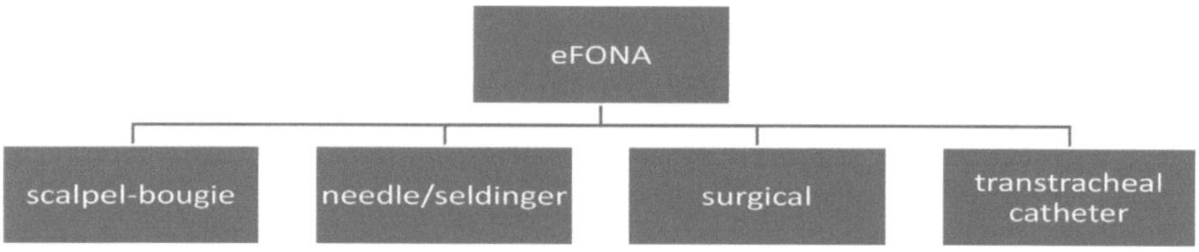

Figure 32.
Approaches for eFONA.

14.1 Scalpel cricothyroidotomy

Using a 'scalpel-bougie-tube' technique is recommended by Difficult Airway Society as the first line technique for eFONA and employs a number 10 blade scalpel, a size 6.0 mm cuffed tracheal tube and a bougie for the same. A 'scalpel-bougie-tube' technique with a horizontal stab incision of the CTM, followed by bougie insertion and rail roading of ETT through the CTM into the trachea is recommended if the CTM is palpable. If this fails, or the CTM is impalpable, then a 8–10 cm vertical incision followed by a 'scalpel-finger-bougie-tube' technique is recommended, wherein blunt dissection with fingers is carried out after skin incision until the CTM is reached, followed by bougie and ETT.

14.2 Needle/seldinger technique

In needle/seldinger technique the trachea is entered with a needle (from commercially available sets) connected to a 5 ml syringe containing 2 ml saline with continuous aspiration, a guidewire passed through it and the cricothyrotomy cannula with its dilator then railroaded over it.

14.3 Surgical technique

The surgical technique involves blunt or scalpel dissection till the CTM, followed by its horizontal incision and passage of the cricothyrotomy cannula (commercially available sets).

14.4 Transtracheal catheter technique

The transtracheal catheter technique similarly involves entering the cricothyroid membrane with a cannula and advancing the transtracheal catheter after needle removal.

Cannulas for these techniques can be narrow bore (ID ≤2 mm) or wide bore (ID ≥4 mm). Narrow bore cricothyroidotomy requires high-pressure ventilation for transtracheal jet ventilation (TTJV) and has drawbacks like misplacement, kinking, and barotrauma. It lacks a tracheal cuff and requires conversion to a definitive airway for aspiration protection and PEEP application. Wide bore cricothyroidotomy's main advantage is enabling conventional ventilation. In the absence of commercial sets, a 14G cannula, a 2 cc syringe barrel, and an 8 mm ETT connector assembly can be used, which can be connected to a breathing circuit or TTJV (**Figure 33**).

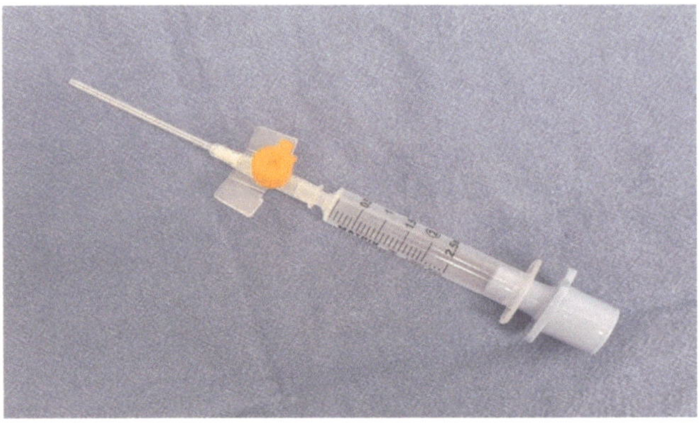

Figure 33.
Transtracheal cricothyrotomy catheter using a 14G cannula,2 cc syringe and 8 mm ETT connector.

15. Airway pharmacology

Airway management, especially endotracheal intubation, requires a deep understanding of airway pharmacology. This procedure can provoke significant physiological responses, like hypertension, tachycardia, increased ICP, and bronchoconstriction. These reactions are usually short-lived but can harm certain patients, such as those with heart disease, cerebral aneurysms, aortic issues, or high blood pressure. Stimulation of the upper airway activates both branches of the autonomic nervous system. In adults, the sympathetic response dominates, increasing catecholamine levels. However, in young children and some adults, it may trigger a vagal response, causing bradycardia. Sedative and hypnotic agents are commonly used to achieve various levels of sedation or anesthesia based on the dose administered [20–22].

The pharmacology of drugs commonly used in emergency airway management are categorized as:

1. Sedative/Hypnotic/Induction agents

2. Muscle Relaxants (Depolarizing and Non-depolarizing Relaxants)

3. Adjunctive Agents

4. Rescue drugs (vasopressors and ionotropes)

5. Neuromuscular Blockade Reversal Agents

16. Post intubation assessment and endotracheal tube care

Confirming endotracheal tube placement traditionally relies on potentially unreliable methods like chest and stomach auscultation (**Table 2**). To ensure reliability, it's recommended to use at least two confirmation methods. The primary choice is ETCO2 detectors, with anteroposterior chest radiography as another option. Fiberoptic bronchoscopy provides a "gold standard" view of tracheal rings, and

Medication	Dose	Onset of action	Duration of action	Physiological effect	Beneficial characteristics	Adverse effects	Major indications
Sedative/hypnotic/induction agents							
Ketamine	0.2–0.5 mg/kg i.v(sedation) 1–2 mg/kg i.v (induction)	1–2 min	5–15 min	↑HR, ↑MAP, ↑$CMRO_2$, ↑ICP, ↑CBF, ↑IOP, ↑Ventilation, Bronchodilation, Analgesia	Bronchodilation, Analgesia	Emergence reaction, Hypertension & Tachycardia, Increases intracranial and intraocular pressures.	Status asthmaticus, Severe hypotension or hypovolaemia
Etomidate	0.2–0.3 mg/kg i.v	30–60 sec	3–5 min	HR(no effect), MAP(no effect), ↓$CMRO_2$, ↓ICP, ↓CBF, ↓Ventilation	Haemodynamic stability	Inhibits cortisol synthesis, monoclonic jerks	CHF, Severe hypotension or hypovolaemia
Propofol	0.25 mg/kg i.v (sedation),1–3 mg/kg i.v (induction)	10–50 sec	3–10 min	↓HR, ↓MAP, ↓$CMRO_2$, ↓ICP, ↓CBF, ↓Ventilation, Bronchodilation	Anticonvulsant effects, Bronchodilation, Suppression of airway reflexes	Respiratory depression, Hypotension, myocardial depression, Pain on injection	Status epilepticus, ↑ICP, Reactive airway disease
Thiopentone sodium	3–5 mg/kg i.v	10–30 sec	5–10 min	↑HR, ↓MAP, ↓$CMRO_2$, ↓ICP, ↓CBF, ↓Ventilation, Bronchoconstriction	Cerebroprotective and Anticonvulsant effects	Hypotension, Myocardial depression, Bronchospasm, Avoid in porphyria	Status epilepticus, ↑ICP
Muscle relaxant/paralytic agents							
Succinylcholine	1.5–2 mg/kg(i.v), 4–5 mg/kg (i.m)	30–60 sec	5–15 min	↑HR (Adults), ↓HR(Children, 2nd dose), ↑IOP	Rapid onset and offset, hence ideal for RSI.	Hyperkalemia, Precipitate malignant hyperthermia Fasciculations,	Essentially all patients except those with: Hyperkalaemia, Causes severe

Medication	Dose	Onset of action	Duration of action	Physiological effect	Beneficial characteristics	Adverse effects	Major indications
						Myalgia, Increase IOP, Bradycardia may occur after repeated doses	hyperkalaemia if used in patients presenting between 5 days-6 months after burns, de-nervation injury, spinal cord injury, stroke
Rocuronium bromide	0.6 mg/kg i.v (allows intubation in 90–120 sec) 1.2 mg/kg, i.v (allows intubation in 60 sec)	60–120 sec	45–70 min	↑HR (at high doses)	Does not have any active metabolites, so better choice for patients requiring prolonged infusions.	Long duration of action	RSI when succinylcholine contraindicated, Rapid reversal with suggamadex.
Atracurium besylate	0.5 mg/kg	90–120 sec	20–45 min	Histamine release can lead to ↓BP & bronchoconstriction	Not metabolized by liver or kidney	Histamine release, Long duration of action	Not recommended for RSI
Vecuronium bromide	0.1–0.3 mg/kg	90–120 sec	45–70 min	Cardiostable	Cardiostable	Long duration of action	Not recommended for RSI
Adjunctive agents							
Lidocaine	1–1.5 mg/kg(i.v)	1–3 mins	~20 mins		Lidocaine will help protect the patient from increases in intracranial pressure, pressor response or cough	Local anesthetic systemic toxicity (if given in high dose)	Head injury, traumatic brain injury, elevated ICP, To be given 2–3 mins before intubation.

DOI: http://dx.doi.org/10.5772/intechopen.1002360

Medication	Dose	Onset of action	Duration of action	Physiological effect	Beneficial characteristics	Adverse effects	Major indications
					reflex to intubation		
Fentanyl	0.5–2 mcg/kg	2–3 min	30–60 min	↓HR, ↓Ventilation	Blunt sympathetic response to intubation, Relatively cardio-stable, Analgesia, Cough suppression	Respiratory depression, chest wall rigidity at high doses	Fentanyl helps decrease catecholamine discharge secondary to intubation,to be given 2–3 mins before intubation.
Midazolam	0.02–0.1 mg/kg i.v (sedation) 0.1–0.4 mg/kg i.v (induction)	2–3 min	15–30 min	↓HR, ↓MAP, ↓$CMRO_2$, ↓ICP, ↓CBF, ↑RR, ↓V_T	Amnesia, Anticonvulsant effects, Relatively cardiostable	Respiratory depression, Long onset, Paradoxical agitation	Status epilepticus
Rescue drugs (vasopressors and ionotropes)							
Ephedrine	Given as boluses of 3 mg i.v	1–2 min	5–10 min	↑HR, ↑CO, ↑BP, ↑Coronary artery blood flow, ↑Myocardial O_2 consumption, ↑RR, Bronchodilation	Direct stimulation of α & β receptors	Tachyphylaxis (usually seen after ~30 mg given), C/I in the presence of MAO inhibitors	Hypotension
Phenylephrine	Given as boluses of 50–100 mcg i.v	< 1 min	5–10 min	↑ BP, ↓HR (reflex)	Direct stimulation of α receptor, ↑coronary pressure without chronotropic effects(useful in cardiac patients)	Bradycardia	Hypotension

Medication	Dose	Onset of action	Duration of action	Physiological effect	Beneficial characteristics	Adverse effects	Major indications
Atropine	0.2–0.6 mg i.v (adult), 20 mcg/kg (children)	< 1 min	20–30 min	↑HR, Bronchodilation, miosis	Antiemetic, Antisialagogue	Crosses BBB causing central anticholinergic syndrome,	Bradycardia, Treatment of organophosphate poisoning.
Neuromuscular blockade reversal agents							
Neostigmine	0.04–0.08 mg/kg i.v	1.5–3 min	4 hrs	↓HR, Bronchoconstriction, ↑ secretions, ↑ peristalsis (mixed with glycopyrolate(0.2 mg per mg of neostigmine) to negate the undesirable cholinergic effects)	Cholinesterase inhibitor	At high doses causes desensitization of post synaptic acetylcholine receptors l/t flaccid paralysis with respiratory failure	Reversal of neuromuscular blockade caused by non-depolarising muscle relaxants
Sugammadex	Moderate block: 2 mg/kg i.v, Deep block: 4 mg/kg i.v, Immediate reversal from RSI: 16 mg/kg i.v			Cardio stable	Reversal of neuromuscular blockade can be performed as quickly as 3 minutes of administration of rocuronium.	Anaphylaxis <1%	Reversal of neuromuscular blockade caused by rocuronium and vecuronium.

Table 2.
Airway pharmacology.

ultrasound can detect tracheal placement and potential unilateral bronchial intubation. Proper endotracheal tube care involves securing it to prevent displacement, maintaining cuff pressure at 25–30 cm H2O to prevent aspiration and air leaks without injuring the airway mucosa, and regular or as-needed suctioning to prevent mucus blockage.

17. Post intubation hypotension (PIH)

Post-intubation hypotension (PIH) is defined as a decrease in systolic blood pressure (SBP) to ≤90 mmHg, a drop of ≥20% from baseline SBP, a decrease in mean arterial pressure (MAP) to ≤65 mmHg, or initiation of vasopressors within 30 minutes post-intubation. Risk factors for PIH include a high pre-intubation shock index, chronic renal disease history, intubation for acute respiratory failure, advanced age, lower MAP before intubation, neuromuscular blockers use, or complications during emergent intubation. To reduce PIH risk, preload with a fluid bolus pre-intubation, use hemodynamically stable drugs like ketamine or reduced-dose etomidate, avoid pretreatment drugs like fentanyl and lidocaine that blunt sympathetic tone, set tidal volume at 6–8 ml/kg with low PEEP, insert a nasogastric tube for stomach decompression, and administer vasopressors before intubation [23].

18. Post intubation cardiac arrest (PICA)

Cardiac arrest within 60 minutes of intubation is a severe complication, alongside failed intubation, esophageal intubation, aspiration, hypoxia, and post-intubation hypotension (PIH). It occurs in about 4% of ER cases with high in-hospital mortality, even after achieving spontaneous circulation. Risk factors include multiple intubation attempts, a high intubation-related shock index (>0.9), neuromuscular blockers use, and pre-intubation vasopressors. Patients may struggle with reduced preload and venous return due to increased intrathoracic pressure during positive pressure ventilation. Additionally, physiological changes in severe diseases like acidosis can worsen with intubation and positive pressure ventilation, while sedatives and neuromuscular blockers inhibit stress-induced catecholamine secretion [23].

19. Special circumstances

19.1 Children

Pediatric airways differ significantly from adults, being narrower, softer, and more prone to obstruction due to smaller anatomy and a different larynx position. Children have a higher risk of rapid desaturation and complications like laryngospasm. To manage their airways effectively, careful assessment, specialized equipment, and techniques are essential. Microcuff endotracheal tubes and length-based resuscitation tapes help determine proper equipment sizes. Children's increased oxygen demand and lower reserve make them vulnerable to rapid hypoxia, especially the younger ones. Avoiding multiple intubation attempts is crucial, and while rapid sequence intubation is effective, awake intubation with retained spontaneous respiration is common in children [24].

19.2 Pregnancy

Airway management in pregnant women is complex due to physiological and anatomical changes that occur during pregnancy (**Table 3**). These changes affect both the technical and physiological aspects of airway management. Laryngoscopy becomes more challenging, and there may be a need for smaller-sized endotracheal tubes. The risks of airway bleeding, desaturation, and aspiration increase. It is crucial to optimize all factors involved to ensure success on the first attempt. The use of a short handle direct laryngoscope may be preferred, and the consideration of a bougie is recommended. Preoxygenation, positioning with a 20-to-30-degree head-up tilt, and apneic oxygenation can help further reduce the risk of desaturation. Additionally, uterine displacement through left lateral tilt can be beneficial in preventing supine hypotension syndrome [25].

19.3 Obesity

Obesity affects airway control by reducing space in the pharyngeal tissues and increasing upper airway resistance. It also leads to restrictive lung disease with decreased functional residual capacity (FRC), lung compliance, and alveolar hypoventilation. To manage obese patients' airways effectively, it's essential to position them with an elevated head before intubation, promoting lung expansion, increasing FRC, and oxygen reserve. For obese patients with obstructive sleep apnea undergoing bariatric surgery, the sitting position is recommended for preoxygenation. Due to their heightened risk of rapid desaturation after anesthesia induction, non-invasive positive pressure ventilation (NIPPV) can be used to enhance preoxygenation and extend desaturation time. Implementing head-elevated preoxygenation is crucial for optimal results [11].

19.4 Elevated intracranial pressure

In patients with suspected elevated intracranial pressure (ICP), improper airway management can lead to secondary brain injury and poor neurological outcomes. To

	Pediatric	**Adult**
Tongue	Relatively larger	Relatively smaller
Larynx	Opposite 2nd & 3rd cervical vertebrae	Opposite 4th & 5th cervical vertebrae
Epiglottis	"U" shaped and short	Spade shaped,flat,erect,flexible
Hyoid/ Thyroid sepration	Very close	Further apart
Glottis	½ cartilage	¼ cartilage
Arytenoids	Inclined inferiorly	Horizontal
Vocal cords	Concave	Horizontal
Cricoid	Plate forms funnel	Plate and vertical
Smaller diameter	Cricoid ring	Vocal cord aperture
Consistency of cartilage	Soft	Firm
Shape of head	Pronounced occiput	Flatter occiput

Table 3.
Differences between pediatric and adult airway.

mitigate ICP increase, rapid sequence intubation (RSI) should prioritize normocapnia, oxygenation, and blood pressure control. Proper choice of induction agents, sedatives, and analgesia is crucial. Maintain a target partial pressure of carbon dioxide (PaCO2) between 35 and 45 mmHg to avoid cerebral vasodilation and elevated ICP. End-tidal CO2 (ETCO2) can guide normocapnia and prevent hypo- or hyperventilation. Hyper-ventilation is a last resort for acute ICP rise. Preoxygenation and bag valve mask ventilation should aim for oxygen saturation above 94%. Lowering the bed's head should be minimal and brief, with post-intubation elevation to at least 30° to aid cerebral venous drainage. Etomidate is suitable for brain injury due to minimal hemodynamic effects, and opioid fentanyl pretreatment helps prevent sympathetic responses. Propofol reduces ICP but can cause hypotension, while ketamine is now considered safe with favorable hemodynamics. Succinylcholine and rocuronium are common neuromuscular blockers; succinylcholine's ICP increase is no longer significant, offering rapid onset and shorter duration, facilitating quicker neurological evaluation. Rocuronium, ideal in hyperkalemia risk, has no known ICP effects [26].

20. Role of ultrasound in airway management

Upper airway ultrasound, as a valuable and noninvasive point-of-care ultrasound (POCUS) technique, offers simplicity, portability, and usefulness in evaluating airway management, even in cases where the anatomy is distorted by pathology or trauma. By visualizing important structures such as the thyroid cartilage, epiglottis, cricoid cartilage, cricothyroid membrane, tracheal cartilages, and esophagus, clinicians gain a better understanding of the applied sonoanatomy. This empowers them to utilize ultrasound for various purposes, including assessing difficult intubation, determining appropriate depths for endotracheal tube (ETT) and laryngeal mask airway (LMA) placement, evaluating airway size, guiding invasive procedures like percutaneous needle cricothyroidotomy and tracheostomy, predicting postextubation stridor, determining the appropriate size for left double-lumen bronchial tubes, and detecting upper airway pathologies [27].

21. Conclusion

In conclusion, airway management is a vital aspect of emergency care that saves lives and minimizes complications. This chapter emphasized a systematic approach to assess airway issues through signs, symptoms, patient history, and examination. It highlighted various intervention techniques, from basic maneuvers to advanced procedures, ensuring a clear airway and adequate oxygenation. Equipment selection, including laryngoscopes, tubes, and adjuncts, was discussed with a focus on understanding their indications and limitations. Continuous training and practice are crucial for maintaining proficiency. This chapter offers a comprehensive overview, equipping professionals with the knowledge and skills to approach emergencies confidently. In summary, airway management is a dynamic field requiring a multidisciplinary approach and strong understanding of assessment, intervention techniques, and equipment use, ultimately improving emergency care and patient outcomes.

Acknowledgements

I express deep gratitude to those who significantly contributed to this chapter. First, I thank my father, Dinesh Kumar Dhir, for his unwavering support and belief in my abilities. To my mother, Neelam Dhir, I appreciate your strength and boundless love. My wife, Sonam Dhir, has been my anchor, and her encouragement fuels my drive for excellence. Dr. Susheela Taxak, my teacher, has been pivotal in my academic growth, and her mentorship is invaluable. I also thank my coauthors Dr. Mayank Dhir and Dr. Garima Jain for their support and feedback. Your contributions shaped my thoughts and ideas. I'm profoundly grateful to all of you for being integral to my journey.

With deep gratitude,

Dr. Gaurav Dhir.

Conflict of interest

The authors declare no conflict of interest.

Appendices and nomenclature

i.v (intravenous), i.m (intramuscular), min (minutes), sec (second), HR (heart rate), MAP (mean arterial pressure), CMRO2 (cerebral metabolic rate of oxygen), ICP (intra cranial pressure), CBF (cerebral blood flow), IOP (intra occular pressure), CHF (congestive heart failure), BP (blood pressure), RR (respiratory rate), VT (tidal volume), CO (cardiac output), BBB (blood brain barrier), RSI (rapid sequence intubation), SGD (supraglottic airway device).

Author details

Gaurav Dhir[1*], Mayank Dhir[2] and Garima Jain[3]

1 Marengo Asia Hospitals, Faridabad, India

2 Emergency Medicine, MNR Medical College, Telangana, India

3 Fortis Hospital, Mohali, India

*Address all correspondence to: gauravdhir2003@gmail.com

References

[1] Goto T, Goto Y, Hagiwara Y, Okamoto H, Watase H, Hasegawa K. Advancing emergency airway management practice and research. Acute Medicine & Surgery. 2019;**6**(4): 336-351. DOI: 10.1002/ams2.428

[2] Chou HC, Wu TL. Large hypopharyngeal tongue: A shared anatomic abnormality for difficult mask ventilation, difficult intubation, and obstructive sleep apnea? Anesthesiology. 2001;**94**:936-937

[3] Benumof JL. Obstructive sleep apnea in the adult obese patient: Implications for airway management. Anesthesiology Clinics of North America. 2002;**20**: 789-811

[4] Isono S. Obesity and obstructive sleep apnoea: Mechanisms for increased collapsibility of the passive pharyngeal airway. Respirology. 2012;**17**:32-42

[5] Weibel ER. Geometry and dimensions of airways of conductive and transitory zones. In: Morphometry of the Human Lung. Berlin, Heidelberg: Springer; 1963. pp. 110-135

[6] Myatra SN, Shah A, Kundra P, Patwa A, Ramkumar V, Divatia JV, et al. All India difficult airway association 2016 guidelines for the management of unanticipated difficult tracheal intubation in adults. Indian Journal of Anaesthesia. 2016;**60**(12):885-898. DOI: 10.4103/0019-5049.195481

[7] Khan RM, Sharma PK, Kaul N. Airway management in trauma. Indian Journal of Anaesthesia. 2011;**55**(5): 463-469. DOI: 10.4103/0019-5049.89870

[8] Rosenberg MB, Phero JC, Becker DE. Essentials of airway management, oxygenation, and ventilation: Part 2: Advanced airway devices: Supraglottic airways. Anesthesia Progress. 2014 Fall; **61**(3):113-118. DOI: 10.2344/0003-3006-61.3.113

[9] Gerstein N, Braude D, Hung O, Sanders J, Murphy M. The Fastrach (TM) intubating laryngeal mask airway (R): An overview and update. Canadian Journal of Anaesthesia = Journal Canadien D'anesthésie. 2010;**57**:588-601. DOI: 10.1007/s12630-010-9272-x

[10] Passi Y, Sathyamoorthy M, Lerman J, Heard C, Marino M. Comparison of the laryngoscopy views with the size 1 miller and Macintosh laryngoscope blades lifting the epiglottis or the base of the tongue in infants and children <2 yr of age†. British Journal of Anaesthesia. 2014;**113**:869-874. DOI: 10.1093/bja/aeu228

[11] Lotia S, Bellamy MC. Anaesthesia and morbid obesity. Continuing Education in Anaesthesia Critical Care & Pain. 2008;**8**(5):151-156. DOI: 10.1093/bjaceaccp/mkn030

[12] Ramkumar V. Preparation of the patient and the airway for awake intubation. Indian Journal of Anaesthesia. 2011;**55**(5):442-447. DOI: 10.4103/0019-5049.89863

[13] Wong DT, Yang JJ, Mak HY, Jagannathan N. Use of intubation introducers through a supraglottic airway to facilitate tracheal intubation: A brief review. Canadian Journal of Anaesthesia. 2012;**59**(7):704-715. DOI: 10.1007/s12630-012-9714-8 Epub 2012 Jun 1

[14] Ehrenfeld JM, Cassedy EA, Forbes VE, Mercaldo ND, Sandberg WS. Modified rapid sequence induction and

intubation: A survey of United States current practice. Anesthesia and Analgesia. 2012;**115**(1):95-101. DOI: 10.1213/ANE.0b013e31822dac35 Epub 2011 Oct 24

[15] Weingart SD. Preoxygenation, reoxygenation, and delayed sequence intubation in the emergency department. The Journal of Emergency Medicine. 2011;**40**(6):661-667. DOI: 10.1016/j.jemermed.2010.02.014 Epub 2010 Apr 8

[16] Sahay N, Samaddar DP, Chatterjee A, Sahay A, Kant S, Ranjan A. Sniff to see. Comparing sniffing position versus simple head extension position for glottic exposure - a prospective, randomized cross over study. Journal of Health Specialties. 2016;**4**:212. DOI: 10.4103/2468-6360.186503

[17] Hassan EA, Baraka AAE. The effect of reverse Trendelenburg position versus semi-recumbent position on respiratory parameters of obese critically ill patients: A randomised controlled trial. Journal of Clinical Nursing. 2021;**30**(7–8): 995-1002. DOI: 10.1111/jocn.15645 Epub 2021 Jan 25

[18] Chiang TL, Tam KW, Chen JT, et al. Non-invasive ventilation for preoxygenation before general anesthesia: A systematic review and meta-analysis of randomized controlled trials. BMC Anesthesiology. 2022;**22**:306. DOI: 10.1186/s12871-022-01842-y

[19] Price TM, McCoy EP. Emergency front of neck access in airway management. BJA Education. 2019; **19**(8):246-253. DOI: 10.1016/j.bjae.2019.04.002 Epub 2019 Jun 14

[20] Consilvio C, Kuschner W, Lighthall G. The pharmacology of airway management in critical care. Journal of Intensive Care Medicine. 2011;**27**: 298-305. DOI: 10.1177/0885066611402154

[21] Lindsay S, Benger J. Pharmacology of emergency airway drugs. In: Burtenshaw A, Benger J, Nolan J, editors. Emergency Airway Management. Cambridge: Cambridge University Press; 2015. pp. 63-79. DOI: 10.1017/CBO9781107707542.009

[22] Ghatehorde NK, Regunath H. Intubation Endotracheal Tube Medications. Treasure Island (FL): StatPearls Publishing; 2023 Available from: https://www.ncbi.nlm.nih.gov/books/NBK459276/

[23] Althunayyan SM. Shock index as a predictor of post-intubation hypotension and cardiac arrest; a review of the current evidence. Bull Emerg Trauma. 2019;7(1): 21-27. DOI: 10.29252/beat-070103

[24] Harless J, Ramaiah R, Bhananker SM. Pediatric airway management. International Journal of Critical Illness and Injury Science. 2014;**4**(1):65-70. DOI: 10.4103/2229-5151.128015

[25] Tolga Saracoglu K, Cakmak G, Saracoglu A. Airway management during pregnancy and labor. In: Special Considerations in Human Airway Management. London, UK: IntechOpen; 2021. DOI: 10.5772/intechopen.96476

[26] Khandelwal A, Bithal PK, Rath GP. Anesthetic considerations for extracranial injuries in patients with associated brain trauma. Journal of Anaesthesiology Clinical Pharmacology. 2019;**35**(3):302-311. DOI: 10.4103/joacp.JOACP_278_18

[27] Osman A, Sum KM. Role of upper airway ultrasound in airway management. Journal of Intensive Care. 2016;**4**:52. DOI: 10.1186/s40560-016-0174-z

Chapter 3

Difficult Airway and Its Management

Nigar Kangarli and Asım Esen

Abstract

In the emergency unit, there may not be enough time for proper airway evaluation of a patient with respiratory distress. However, albeit fast, evaluation of head and neck mobility, lower jaw position, condition of teeth, mouth opening, mouth anatomy, and jaw-thyroid distance can contribute significantly to the correct management of the process. Based on these results, a decision can be made on how to manage the airway and how to proceed. If there is a finding of a difficult airway, a call for help should not be delayed. Ready-to-use "emergency airway management kit" is important. Determining whether the condition is a "difficult airway" is important because the "anticipated difficult airway" and "unanticipated difficult airway" approaches are different. There are numerous options for providing respiratory support to patients, and conservative approaches should be prioritized. Definitely, in addition to respiratory support with bag-masks, supraglottic airway devices, endotracheal tubes, and tracheostomy approach may also be processed without delay, in case of need. The aim of all procedures is to provide the patient with oxygen, which is indispensable for life. It should not be forgotten to avoid oxygen neglection during selecting the method, which requires least interventions and guarantees airway security. Consequently, in semi-urgent states, a more detailed evaluation of the patient is more appropriate.

Keywords: difficult airway, airway management, emergency medicine, 'can't intubate can't oxygenate', airway ultrasound

1. Introduction

Secured airway is the cornerstone of effective resuscitation at life-threating states. Emergency practitioners are at the frontline for resuscitation of complex situations when airway management is far different from that in elective conditions. The shortage of time for decision-making and diagnosing the pathologic state also contributes to management failure.

It is important for practitioners to be aware and prepared for complicated intubation situations to reduce unpleasant outcomes and to provide high-quality healthcare. This chapter is aimed to discuss difficult airway prediction and the most used airway management devices and offers easy-to-understand descriptions of instrumentation techniques. Among the predictive difficult airway parameters, this chapter covers a brief explanation of ultrasound guided methods to foresee the airway complexity. The manuscript also contains revised guidelines for difficult airway management, accepted worldwide, and includes suggestions for specific complicated airway circumstances. We hope this chapter's content would be helpful for airway managers in complicated circumstances and beneficial to improve the outcomes.

2. Definitions

Difficult airway (DA) is one of the most frightening situations, which may possibly be faced by practitioners in emergency, intensive care departments, and operating rooms. Inability to secure airway increases mortality associated with hypoxic brain injury and cardiopulmonary arrest. The core definition of DA was adopted by The American Society of Anesthesiologists (ASA) as the clinical situation in which a conventionally trained anesthesiologist has trouble with face mask ventilation of the upper airway, difficulty with tracheal intubation, or both [1]. Both these definitions may be uncovered and classified further into separate variations. Here, we encounter the most common variations of difficult airway conditions.

2.1 Difficult face mask ventilation

Authors define this condition as the inability of an experienced specialist (intensivist or anesthesiologist) to maintain oxygen saturation above 90% with a 100% FiO2 face mask [2]. The condition occurs generally as a consequence of inadequate mask seal, excessive gas leak (both are seen mainly in patients with complicated face anatomy, obesity, age over 65, "no teeth," and beard and/or mustache), or excessive resistance to gas inflow and outflow (seen in cases with "stiff lungs" or foreign body in the airways).

2.2 Difficult supraglottic airway ventilation

Difficult supraglottic airway ventilation is defined the same as difficult face mask ventilation and occurs in the same circumstances.

2.3 Difficult supraglottic airway placement

Difficult supraglottic airway placement encounters the inability to place supraglottic device after multiple attempts in the presence or absence of tracheal pathology.

2.4 Difficult tracheal intubation

Difficult tracheal intubation is a state of unsuccessful tracheal tube placement after three or more attempts or time elapse more than 10 minutes spent to perform tracheal tube placement by due to presence or absence of tracheal pathology. Difficult tracheal intubation (orotracheal, nasotracheal, or transtracheal) may occur as the consequence of difficult laryngoscopy (inability to visualize any portion of vocal cords after multiple attempts) or failed intubation (incorrect placement of the intubation tube after multiple attempts).

2.5 Difficult surgical transtracheal intubation

Difficult surgical transtracheal intubation covers the terms of unsuccessful cricothyrotomy or tracheotomy after multiple attempts processed by skilled practitioner [2, 3].

3. Prediction

Proper physical examination and medical history of a patients may provide clues for prediction of DA. It is important for practitioners to be aware and prepared for complicated intubation situations to reduce unpleasant outcomes and to provide high-quality healthcare. Depending on whether the cases are predicted to be difficult or not, airways are classified into anticipated and unanticipated. As a common rule, not all anticipated difficult airways appear problematic at performance. Emergency department practitioners do not generally have enough time for detailed physical examination of a patient with the risk of respiratory collapse. However, a quick look on patient's overall appearance may be profitable. Examination in elective circumstances starts with head and neck assessment and includes:

3.1 The jaw opening

In general, it is about 4 cm, which could be easily measured by three finger breadths between upper and lower incisors. The jaw opening lesser that three fingers is considered as limited mouth opening and complicates laryngoscope blade positioning in the mouth.

3.2 Size of the tongue

It is usually examined during the evaluation of Mallampati score. Extremely large tongues in contrast to mouth diameter are also predisposed to DA.

3.3 Abnormal teeth or lack of teeth

Incomplete frontal dentition, presence of loose teeth or prosthesis, inappropriate prognation (inability to protrude the mandible so that the lower incisors are anterior to the upper incisors), and too prominent upper incisors.

3.4 Abnormal congenital or acquired mandibular anatomy

Micrognathia (small size of mandible) and retrognathia (abnormally posterior location of mandible compared to maxilla) are two main structural abnormalities of mandibular shape, which are predisposed to DA. These rare conditions occur 1 in 1500 live births worldwide [4, 5] and are generally associated with inborn genetic errors, for instance, Pierre Robin sequence, Treacher Collins syndrome, branchio-oculo-facial syndrome, cri du chat syndrome, trisomy 13 and trisomy 18, and so on [6]. Acquired mandibular or maxilla pathologies are commonly associated with maxillofacial traumas and burns.

3.5 Head and neck mobility

Cervical range of motion decreases with age. Cervical spine arthritis, ankylosing spondylitis, previous cervical surgery, and neck collar presence due to traumatic accident may lead to restricted neck extension, which complicates the positioning of head for successful intubation.

3.6 Neck circumference

Normal values are <37 cm in males and < 34 cm in females. Obesity, thyroid gland diseases, obstructive sleep apnea syndrome, and pregnancy are among the most common reasons of increased neck circumference.

3.7 Presence of facial hair, beard

The presence of beard or moustache predisposes to difficulties with mask sealing during ventilation and air leak through facial hair.

3.8 Mallampati classification

It was described in 1985 as a test to predict difficult laryngoscopy and involves the assessment of how far the tongue size restricts pharyngeal view.

- Class I: Tonsillar pillars, uvula, and hard and soft palates are easily visualized.
- Class II: Partial uvula and soft palate are visualized.
- Class III: Only the soft palate is visualized.
- Class IV: No uvula or soft palate is visualized.

3.9 Cormack-Lehane (CL) score

It was described in 1984. This score, unfortunately, has little correlation with Mallampati score, so it is impossible to predict the CL grade by simple physical examination of the patient. CL is assessed only after direct laryngoscopy has been proceeded and is expressed as the degree of glottis aperture visualization. The updated CL description is as follows:

- Grade 1: A full view of glottis including arytenoid cartilages, vocal cords, and epiglottis.
- Grade 2a: Only posterior laryngeal aperture is visualized and includes part of vocal cords, arytenoids, and epiglottis.
- Grade 2b: Posterior aperture and vocal cords are not visualized; only arytenoids are defined.
- Grade 3: Only epiglottis is visualized (no vocal cords, no arytenoids).
- Grade 4: No glottis structure is visualized (no epiglottis, no vocal cords, no arytenoids).

Both Mallampati and CL scores > 3 are considered as difficult laryngoscopy and intubation circumstances and require difficult airway preparation.

3.10 Upper lip bite test (ULBT)

Sensitivity of ULBT in prediction of DA is more than 70%. Specificity for ULBT is >85% [7]. Upper lip bite test evaluates mandibular movement, which is important during tongue root elevation with laryngoscope blade. To measure the mandibular joint mobility, the patients are asked to bite their upper lip with lower incisors as high as they can [8].

- Class I: Lower incisors can bite above the vermilion border of the upper lip.
- Class II: Lower incisors cannot reach vermillion border.
- Class III: Lower incisor cannot bite upper lip.

3.11 Thyromental distance

It is the distance between thyroid notch and chin tip. Normal range is fluctuative, depending on the age and gender, but measurements <6.5 cm (3 finger breadths) indicate anticipated DA.

3.12 Hyomental distance

It is the distance between hyoid bone and chin tip. Normal range is equal or more than 4 cm (2 finger breadths). Distance less than two fingers is predisposed to DA.

3.13 3-3-2 rule

It is a simple tool for difficult intubation prediction, which combines three distinct measurements: three finger breadths between upper and lower incisors, three finger breadths between thyroid notch and chin, and two finger breadths between hyoid cartilage and chin. The distances should not be measured in head-extended position!

3.14 LEMON

It is an abbreviation of another difficult intubation prediction tool, which is extremely useful and quick. The higher the score, the harder is the intubation. This method was first developed by Scottish emergency department practitioners after evaluating data from patients diagnosed with anticipated difficult airways, between June 2002 and September 2003 [9].

L-look externally:	
facial trauma	1 point
large incisors	1 point
beard or mustache	1 point
large tongue	1 point

E-evaluate the 3-3-2 rule:	
interincisor distance 3 finger breadths	1 point
thyromental distance 3 finger breadths	1 point
hyomental distance 2 finger breadths	1 point
M-Mallampati score > 3	1 point.
O-obstruction (may be quickly suspected if stridor is present)/obesity	1 point
N-neck mobility (asking the patient for cervical extension and flexion/ presence of collar or any other evident neck immobility feature)	1 point

3.15 Six features have been identified as likely to cause difficulty with bag mask ventilation (BMV)

- Presence of beard
- Lack of teeth
- Age > 55
- BMI > 30
- History of snoring
- Inability to protrude mandible

3.16 MOANS

The potential DA predictive features were further incorporated into MOANS mnemonic by American Emergency Airway Course:

- M-mask seal (ineffective due to presence of beard, blood, trauma)
- O-obesity/obstruction
- A-age
- N-no teeth
- S-stiff lungs

No single tool or assessment method was identified as consistently being more predictive than another, and multivariate measures intended to predict difficult airway were too few and diverse among the studies to determine a common list of predictors [3]. Experience confirms that a better way to judge on the severity of airway difficulty of a patient is to interpret the anatomical and physiological features in combination, naturally in the presence of sufficient time interval.

4. Using ultrasound guidance (USG) for evaluation

Even after using multiple clinical screening tests, a significant incidence of unanticipated difficult laryngoscopy (1–8%) has been observed [10]. In addition, the clinical assessment tools play a limited role in unconscious and uncooperative individuals [11]. So, in addition to general data, based on facial features, anatomical landmarks, and measurements, we would like to share a brief overview of measurements obtained from ultrasonography inspection of a patient. There are plenty of distance measurements between significant head and neck landmarks that provide foresight concerning the degree of being at loss of airway management. Ultrasound usage in all departments and among practitioners has become extremely widespread, and there seems to be no obstacle for emergency doctors to evaluate several features in elective circumstances. According to the 2022 ASA Practice Guideline Difficult Airway Management, measuring the skin-to-hyoid distance, skin-to-epiglottis distance, and tongue volume by USG is the simplest, fastest, and most sufficient way to decide whether the airway is complicated or not.

4.1 Skin-to-epiglottis distance (DSE)

In the absence of front neck adipose tissue, this distance is the same as skin-to-thyrohyoid membrane distance (DST). This distance is the most predictive and trusted among USG measurements. The distance may be measured in parasagittal or mid-transverse plane. Is also measured with linear probe placed sagittal (**Figure 1**) or transversely (**Figure 2**) over the midway between hyoid bone and thyroid cartilage

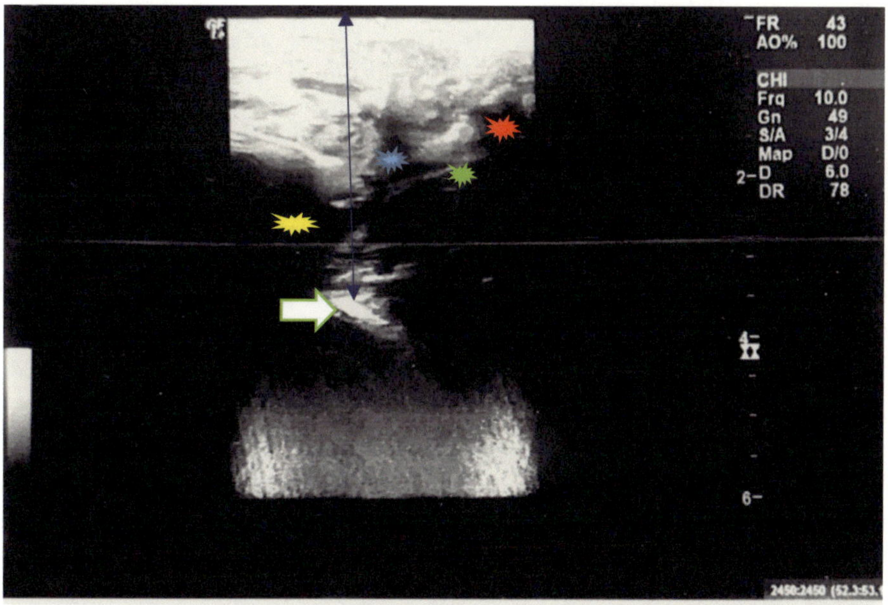

Figure 1.
Parasagittal USG view of DSE. Blue star: hyoid bone, red star: thyroid cartilage, green star: thyrohyoid membrane, yellow star: tongue root, white arrow: epiglottis, blue arrow: DSE. Copyright belongs to the authors.

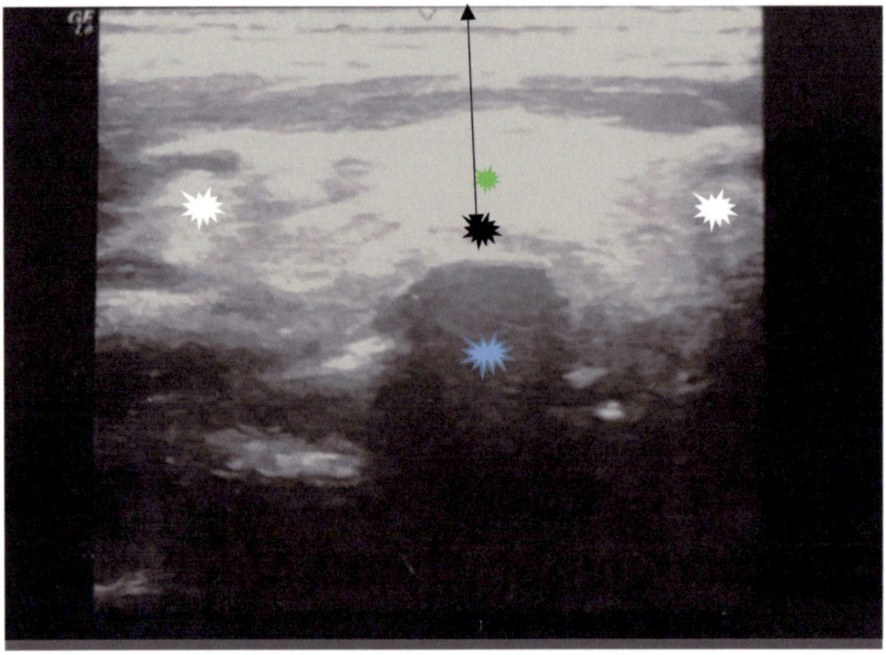

Figure 2.
Transverse USG view of DSE. Green star: pre-epiglottic space, white stars: sternocleidomastoid muscles, black star: epiglottis, blue star: glottis, black arrow: DSE. Copyright belongs to the authors.

(at the level of the epiglottis). Epiglottis is identified as a curvilinear hypoechoic structure with a bright posterior air mucosal interface and hyperechoic pre-epiglottic space. It is important to mention that this distance shows variations in men and women, so there is no clearly defined value. According to Guan et al. [12], a cutoff value of 2.36 cm was optimized for DSE and proved to be more powerful predictive value than other USG indicators for predicting a difficult laryngoscopy. This research points on high sensitivity of 95% and specificity of 95% of DSE as an independent predictive feature. Pinto et al. [13] evaluated the use of the USG measured distance from the skin to epiglottis in the transverse plane and demonstrated that a cutoff value of 2.75 cm was effective for classifying easy versus difficult laryngoscopies. Falcetta et al. [14] also measured this same distance and found that a cutoff value of 2.54 cm was the most effective. The larynx is usually higher in males than in females; on the other hand, laryngoscopy during intubation leads to manual elevation of epiglottis, and consequently, the distance measured prior to instrumentation now becomes shorter. To abolish doubts on eligibility and accuracy of DSE measurement, the parasagittal measurement is recommended, as it avoids the effect of a high larynx and can clearly visualize the adjoining relationship with the various larynx structures. Another research on DSE, conducted by Chabbra et al. [15] in 2022, defines the cutoff value of > 1.67 cm to predict difficult laryngoscopy (the study encounters measurements in mid-transverse plane at the level of vocal cords) but with lower sensitivity (64.71%) and specificity (78.45%). Resuming all the mentioned above, the approximate cutoff >2.36 cm is strongly associated with CL > grade 3 during parasagittal measurements; a cutoff >1.67 cm is suspicious of CL > grade 2 during transverse measurements.

4.2 Skin-to-hyoid distance (DSH)

It is measured by placing the linear high-frequency US probe transversely over the hyoid cartilage. The hyoid cartilage is visualized as a curved echogenic lining with posterior acoustic shadow (**Figure 3**). According to Wu et al. [16], the distance more than 1.28 cm predicts a difficult laryngoscopy.

4.3 Tongue volume

It is measured by a low-frequency convex probe with the patient in supine position with head extended, mouth closed, and tongue slightly touching the incisors (**Figure 4**). The probe is placed under the chin in the median sagittal plane and adjusted to obtain the entire tongue outline clearly on the screen. The maximal vertical dimension from the tongue surface to the skin is measured as the tongue thickness. Although no clear data on cutoff value of tongue thickness exists, significant study was conducted by Andruskiewicz's et al. [17], and tongue volumes >12 cm show correlation with difficult laryngoscopy and difficult intubation.

5. Preparation and equipment

The main goal during management of anticipated or unanticipated difficult airway cases is to provide sufficient oxygenation. Time losses on decision-making, unsuccessful attempts, or equipment supply should not cause an interruption in the oxygen supply to the tissues. Remember, the goal is to provide ventilation, for

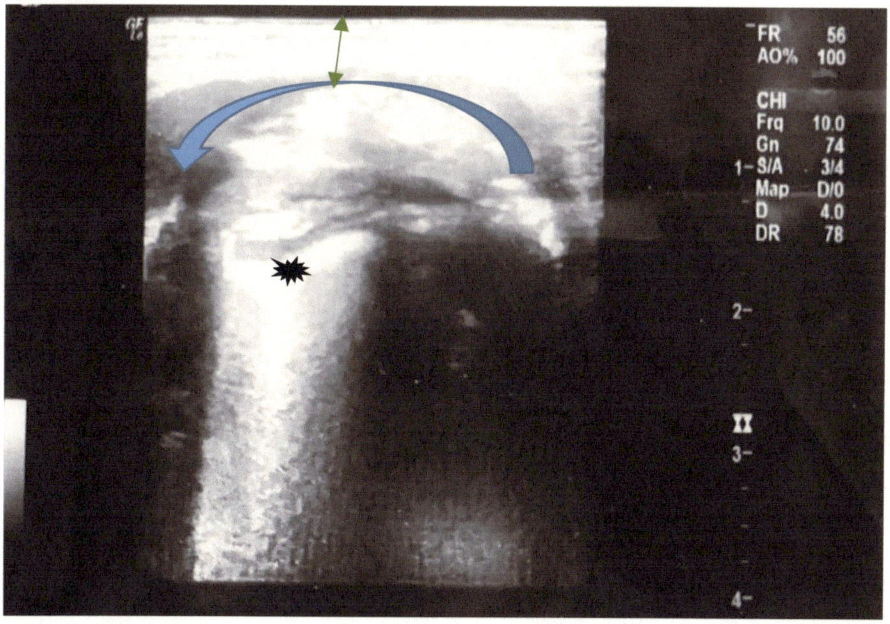

Figure 3.
Transverse US view of DSH. Black star: Epiglottis, blue arrow: Hyoid bone, green arrow: DSH. Copyright belongs to the authors.

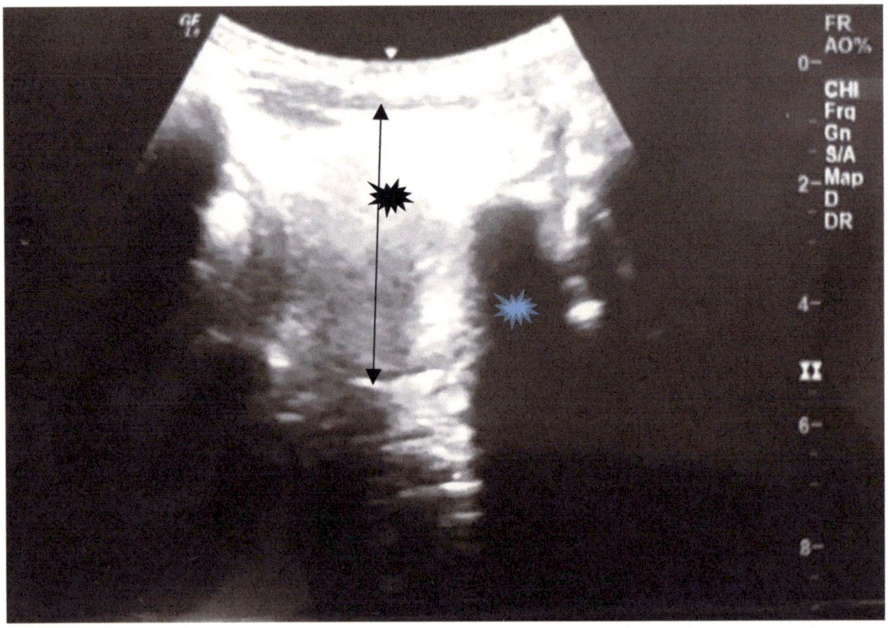

Figure 4.
Tongue volume USG measurement. Black star: tongue, black arrow: tongue volume, blue star: hyoid bone. Copyright belongs to the authors.

example, inflow and outflow of fresh gas in order to sustain tissue metabolism. It is not exactly intubation or any other invasive airway access that saves the lives. As it is known, oxygenation is of vital importance. In cases when laryngoscopy and endotracheal intubation seems difficult, and BMV provides necessary oxygenation, it is wiser to simply ventilate the victim in spite of losing time on unsuccessful intubation attempts. If DA is known or strongly suspected:

- Ensure the presence of difficult airway cart or emergency trolley with difficult airway equipment.
- Call for help as soon as possible. Do not struggle on DA or pursue intubation rather than calling for assistance or maintaining oxygenation.
- Airway management should be performed by the most skilled practitioner in the field.
- Make sure to provide the most proper position that will ease instrumentation and ventilation.
- Capnography should be used wherever airway performance is undertaken to confirm correct airway device placement. If there is CO2 in the exhaled air, the endotracheal tube (ETT) is in the trachea, and capnography is considered the "gold standard" in this respect. Do not forget: "no Trace=wrong Place" [18].
- Strictly administer supplemental oxygen before initiating airway management, and keep delivering whenever feasible throughout the whole process.

- If CICO ("can't intubate can't oxygenate"-the situation when failed intubation is compounded by the inability to maintain adequate oxygen saturation with BMV) diagnosed, surgical airway must be performed immediately.

Where difficult airways are anticipated, management includes the following basic attitudes and interventions:

5.1 Airway maneuvers

The most commonly used airway manipulation is backward-upward rightward pressure (BURP) adjustment on the larynx, performed externally by repositioning thyroid cartilage, and the best laryngeal view is obtained to assist intubation. Another maneuver is external cricoid pressure (Sellick maneuver), used for proper visualization of vocal cords. Appropriate head and neck position is also important for successful airway management. The aim of Sniffing position, which is broadly used among anesthesiologists and emergency practitioners, is to bring the laryngeal and pharyngeal axes as close as possible to the oral axis. The position is easily given after placement of 10 cm pillow under patient's occipital bone and involves cervical flexion and head extension. The "jaw thrust chin lift" is a principal and extremely trusted maneuver practiced among anesthesiologist. The simultaneous chin protrusion and elevation, achieved by mandibular angle manipulation with dominant single hand or both hands, mostly requires a second person and improves BMV in almost all cases.

5.2 Noninvasive airway management devices

In case of anticipated DA, it is important to adequately preoxygenate the patient, to earn extra time during airway management attempts. Preoxygenation increases oxygen reserves (saturation of forced reserve lung capacity is especially important in pediatric cases, who are extremely predisposed to desaturation after even subtle apnea period) and delays the onset of hypoxia, and this way allows time for rescue instrumentations. In anesthesiology practice, we prefer the term denitrogenation as a synonym for preoxygenation, as not only oxygen reserve is fulfilled but also nitrogen present in the residual and reserve lung volumes is replaced with oxygen. Classically, preoxygenation is considered as 3–5 minutes of $FiO2 = 100\%$ patient ventilation at the tidal volumes. This time lag is enough to remove nitrogen from respiratory system. The ASA suggests other versions of preoxygenation. In a case of spontaneously breathing patient (preoxygenation prior to awake intubation), 4–12 breaths at forced vital capacity in 1 minute or shortest time lag with $FiO2 = 100\%$ is enough to avoid desaturation. If FiO2 is possible to be measured (in cases of emergency room air BMV), 3 minutes of oxygen administration to reach an end-tidal oxygen concentration of 0.90 or higher ($EtO2 > 0.9$) is considered an appropriate preoxygenation [3]. The duration of apnea without desaturation can also be prolonged by passive oxygenation (which means the patient shows no spontaneous breathing) during the apneic period. This issue is called apneic oxygenation and can be achieved by administering up to 15 L/min oxygen through nasal cannula [2]. High-flow ventilation devices are used for this purpose and are widely administered for awake intubation, which will be described later. Any healthcare practitioner should be familiar with the basic equipment required for airway management:

5.2.1 Rigid laryngoscopic blades

Macintosh (curved) and Miller (straight) blades are available in sizes from neonatal (No. 0) to large adult (No. 4). The aim of a blade is to remove oral anatomical structures to provide the vision of the glottis. Levering of blades (using shorter or longer blade during intubation attempts) has shown to rise the intubation success rate [3]. As a common rule, straight blades are used for infant intubation, while curved blades are more practicable for adult and pediatric instrumentations.

5.2.2 Adjuncts

Bougies are rubber, elastic, 50–60 cm long wires with 30 degrees angulated tips. They are usually indicated in cases of CL grade 3–4, and the practitioner inserts the bougie just below the epiglottis without seeing the vocal cords. After that, endotracheal tube is inserted over the bougie. Some of them may have lumen and fenestrated tips, so oxygenation may be allowed while providing necessary airway manipulation resources or conducting surgical airway. Some of these devices are equipped with a video or fiber-optic display element at the distal end. Light wands allow the practitioner to view the glottis from outside the mouth; at the same time, the progression of the device through the vocal cords results in light transillumination in the midline of the neck, which confirms proper positioning.

5.2.3 Supraglottic airway devices (SAD)

Laryngeal Mask airways, or so-called LMAs, were first described in 1983 by Archie Brain [2] and are considered one of the milestones of airway management. Additionally, SAD[1] is indicated for CL grade 3–4 cases and difficult BMV situations. Being placed blindly, none of SADs directly intubate the patient but seal around and above the glottis. Thus, they carry the risk of aspiration. Another disadvantage of using LMA is its instability and displacement risk during transportation, even if accurately secured and fixed. The diversity of LMA modifications is now present. Intubating laryngeal mask airway (ILMA), or so-called FASTRACH, has a handle and is used for blind intubations. The sealing mechanism is the same as for classic LMA, whereas FASTRACH has its own special endotracheal tube. Despite blind insertion of the tube, proper tracheal intubation rates are extremely high. The Air-Q Intubating Laryngeal Airway (ILA) was first introduced by Daniel Cook in 2005. It is available in distinct sizes, in both disposable and reusable forms. The only difference from FASTRACH is the absence of a handle. A special intubation tube is inserted, as in the case of ILMA, blindly through the Air-Q. I-Gel LMA is different from mentioned devices in the way its hypopharyngeal part (the part that seals onto the larynx) has a preshaped soft thermoplastic elastomer and has no inflatable cuff, so easier insertion and less trauma is encountered. Except this advantages, I-Gels have gastric channel for aspiration. Recommended insertion depth and size, correlated with weight, are shown on the outer surface of the device.

[1] The SAD are briefly described in this chapter, without detailing, as they are the scope of another chapter.

5.2.4 Retroglottic airway devices (RAD)

Combitube is a double lumen tube, advocated for blind intubations. The tube has two separate lumens: one for esophageal intubation, with single pore at its tip (clear) and another, with multiple fenestrations on both sides, for air entrance into supraglottic area (blue). Esophageal lumen is inflated with 10–15 ml of air and the supraglottic one with 80–100 ml of air. This device is not used in pediatric patients and is present only in two sizes. 37F size is appropriate for patients <170 cm height, and 41F is indicated for patients >170 cm height. The recommended maximum duration for Combitube persistence in the airway is 8 hours. In some cases, blind insertion of Combitube may accidentally intubate trachea, which is not fatal but even beneficial. In this case, just inflating the cuff of the esophageal lumen is enough, just as with ETTs. However, the cases of tracheal intubation with Combitube should definitely be recognized, as the cuff inflation with 10–15 is hazardous for tracheal wall. Separate ventilation of every lumen in combination with midaxillary line lung auscultation is the simplest way to differentiate whether esophagus or trachea is intubated. If respiratory sounds are achieved during ventilation through esophageal lumen (clear one), tracheal intubation should be suspected.

5.2.5 King laryngeal tube (King LT)

It differs from Combitube by having a single pilot balloon for both cuff inflations. This device also has two lumens, both ending up in two apertures: the shorter one beveled anteriorly and the longer one beveled posteriorly. The posteriorly beveled tip of the longer lumen escapes tracheal insertion. This tip should enter esophagus with its smaller cuff preventing regurgitation. Beveled tip allows aspiration catheter insertion through the device and gastric matter aspiration if needed. The shorter lumen has no side fenestrations (in contrast to Combitube), and its anteriorly beveled tip remains just superior to glottis, thus providing laryngopharyngeal ventilation. Esophageal lumen cuff (the smaller one) is inflated inside the esophagus, while the larger supraglottic cuff separates pharynx from larynx just beneath the root of the tongue. As mentioned, both cuffs are inflated by single pilot balloon with 60–100 ml of air, depending on the device size. The size and required air inflation volumes are indicated on the outer side of the tube and accord to patients' height. King LT maximum airway persistence period is the same as for Combitube and is also not recommended for use in children.

The contraindications for Combitube and King LT include obstructive masses or foreign bodies in laryngopharynx, known lesions of esophagus and larynx (as cuff inflation may lead to perforation) and patients with preserved gag reflex. In contrast to supraglottic devices, these ones reduce the risk of airway aspiration and regurgitation.

5.2.6 Videolaryngoscopes

These are preferred in cases when direct laryngoscopy does not provide necessary visualization of glottis. It has more angled blades, a camera built into the blade tip, and a screen. The screen is located on the handle in some and as a separate unit in others. The more angulated blade curvature, in combination with localization of optic camera on the tip of the videolaryngoscope blade, improves the view of glottis aperture. Besides this, ETT insertion and progression in patients with micrognathia or incomplete mouth opening is comforted, as tube passage through the airway is visualized from outside the mouth. Videolaryngoscopes improve Cormack-Lehane views of the larynx by one to two grades [19]. This device should be preferred as first—to pass in high aspiration risk patients. There are two types of videolaryngoscopes: channeled-guided (examples include Airtraq, King Vision, and Pentax) and non-channeled-guided (Glidescope, C-MAC, and McGrath). The difference is that channeled ones are more angulated at the curvature and also have a conduit for ETT guidance (which is beneficial in patients with immobile cervical spine) [19].

5.2.7 Fiberoptic (FBO) intubation and awake airway management

Visualization of airway passage is possible with a flexible endoscope with an optic fiber inside it. The tip of the device is manipulated by a handle from outside the airway. The endotracheal tube is seated along the scope. After proper glottis visualization, the ETT is forwarded to the trachea; then, the fiber optic guide is removed. Insertion of fiberscope may be through nostrils (inferior concha) or through the oral cavity. This technique is appropriate for awake or mildly sedated patients. The reason for this is necessity of tongue and airway wall tonus to be preserved, as fiberscope advancement through collapsed airway restricts reaching the trachea. Awake patient intubation is a complicated but, at the same time, a very safe method to be tracked at elective anticipated difficult airway circumstances. This method is of little practice in emergency departments but anyway deserves a brief discussion. The indications for awake fiberoptic airway intubation include: patients with previously recorded difficult intubation or difficult ventilation history (known CICO cases), predicted difficult airways due to inability to access pre-cricoid or pre-thyroid region, known aspiration risk, and cervical spine immobility.

At the other end, definite contraindications are present:

- Impending airway obstruction (epiglottitis or any other upper airway infection or abscess that may rupture or progress).

- Blood, infection or fragile tumoral tissue in the upper airways (due to potential contamination of lower airways).

- Patient refusal or uncooperative patient.

- Penetrating eye injuries.

- Fractured skull base (accidental fiberoptic device insertion into brain).

- Absence of skilled practitioner.

An important step in the preparation for awake intubation is topical anesthesia. Topical anesthesia can be provided either through surface analgesia or using appropriate nerve blocks [20]. The average dose necessary for topical anesthesia is 8–9 mg/kg lignocaine. It is important to anesthetize oral cavity (or nasal cavity in cases of nasal intubation), pharynx, and larynx. Lignocaine sprays for oral cavity and swabs lubricated with lignocaine for nasal cavity require 5–10 minutes for the top numbness to be achieved. Pharynx is anesthetizes by introducing lignocaine swabs into palatoglossal and palatopharyngeal folds or, simply, by asking the patient to gargle

2% viscous lignocaine. To anesthetize the laryngeal region, injection of lignocaine through cricothyroid membrane in caudad orientation at the end of patient's deep inspiration. This approach causes cough reflex, which ultimately improves the dispersion of local anesthetic. It is important to provide oxygen supply (the most preferred method is high-flow oxygen cannula) during the whole process of topicalization and fiberoscope advancement. The performer may also use the "spray and go" technique: when local anesthetic is injected through fiberoscope's suction canal and oxygen supply is attached to the canal simultaneously. This provides both, oxygenation and topicalization. Successful topicalization may not always be achieved and, besides, takes a little longer time, so practitioners prefer to combine local anesthetic infiltration with light sedation, without neuromuscular blocker addition, as mentioned above, to secure airway tonus for scope fibers progression.

5.3 Invasive airway management techniques

5.3.1 Retrograde wire-guided intubation

This technique includes endotracheal tube progression along a wire, inserted retrograde from the larynx up to the oral cavity. The approach may be considered in cases of oral, pharyngeal, or laryngeal tumors (impossibility of glottis visualization); patients with stiff laryngeal wall (unable to be elevated with laryngoscope blade); unsuccessful intubation attempts; patients with immobile cervical spine due to variety of reasons (ankylosing spondylitis, cervical collar etc.); and especially patients with maxillofacial trauma and burns. A 16–20 G needle is used to puncture the cricothyroid membrane. Care should be taken to avoid thyroid gland, cricothyroid artery, and posterior laryngeal wall damage during puncture. The needle is initially approached 90 degrees to the skin, and negative pressure applied by the syringe. Air rush into the syringe informs that needle is inside the larynx, and at this step, the needle should be redirected 45 degrees cephalad. The guide-wires incorporated into central vein catheterization kits are most commonly used for retrograde intubation. The guide wire is introduced through the needle until it appears out of the mouth or nostrils. Endotracheal intubation tube exchanger (ETT exchanger) is then advanced upon the guide wire, until resistance is felt as anterior laryngeal wall is contacted. At this step, the cephalad end of the guide is exerted with simultaneous advance of ETT exchanger, which consequently passes through vocal cords. The next step is the progression of appropriate sized intubation tube along the exchanger and final drawing out of the ETT exchanger. Do not hesitate BMV, passive oxygenation, or high-flow nasal cannula ventilation of the patient during retrograde airway management! In the case of absence of ETT exchanger, intubation tube may be simply advanced through wire guide, but this method carries risk of tube dislodgement into esophagus or tube clinging at any level throughout the passageway (as the guide wire is too thin to properly route the tube, bigger than self-diameter).

5.3.2 Front-of-neck percutaneous needle cricothyrotomy

The technique resembles the retrograde intubation, except the guide wire is protruded downward into the trachea instead of upwards. Ready kits are present to perform cricothyrotomy. The main goal is to perform a tiny longitudinal incision on the cricothyroid membrane. Then, a needle is inserted into the airway through the incision (again with a negative pressure syringe, and stop advancing as air fills the syringe). The kit needle usually has a plastic catheter over it. Taking care not to puncture the opposite laryngeal wall, the needle is then removed with simultaneous pushing the catheter in caudad direction. A guide wire is introduced; then, the plastic apparatus is removed. Special dilatator present in the kit is slid along the guide with rotational manipulations, again, with care not to harm the opposite wall. After the dilatator is removed, the cannula is introduced through the guide, and the guide finally removed. Both retrograde intubation and cricothyrotomy (as well as tracheotomy) necessitate immobility of thyroid cartilage and laryngeal structures during needle insertion. This is best achieved by fixating the thyroid cartilage with nondominant hand in the following matter: the thumb and middle finger grasp the thyroid cartilage at both sides, thus stabilizing it and preventing movement. Index finger is placed on the cricothyroid membrane, exactly at the point where the needle is inserted (this fixation method is called laryngeal handshake).

5.3.3 Front-of-neck scalpel cricothyrotomy

This method is preferred in cases when no crycothyrotomy kit is available. Depending on whether the cricothyroid membrane is palpable or not (cases of irradiated neck, when the tough front neck tissues are impossible to differentiate), two methods are described in literature. If cricothyroid membrane is easily identified by laryngeal handshake motion, a transverse 4 cm incision is made; blind finger dissection of subcutaneous tissues is performed until the cricothyroid membrane is palpated or visualized. Then, another horizontal incision is made over the membrane itself. Finger palpation of cricoid cartilage and tracheal lumen, together with the incised aperture dilatation, assists the bougie (or 6.0 mm ETT tube) insertion in caudad orientation at the depth less than 10 cm (carina is reached at that depth). Then, the 6.0 mm ETT is slid along the bougie into the airways. If cricothyroid membrane is not palpated properly, a vertical incision is preferred. It may extend upward until mandibula or downward until sternum in order to anatomically define the membrane.

5.3.4 Front-of-neck percutaneous tracheostomy

Out of scope of emergency airway management.

6. Guidelines

The steps, which should be followed in cases of difficult airway, were described by American Association of Anesthesiology (ASA) and Difficult Airway Society (DAS) [21]. First DAS guideline was adopted in 2015, and the recommendations are repeatedly updated and revised. Here, we submit 2022 difficult intubation guideline, as the simplest way to decide on which action to choose (**Figures 5** and **6**).

During Plan A, if the laryngoscopy is unsuccessful, return back to ventilation and suggest which maneuvers may challenge your laryngoscopy. Reposition patient's head, administer paralytic drug (in cases when vocal cords are visible, but intubation is made impossible due to their closed state), use external maneuvers, discussed above, and try laryngoscopy again. A max of 3 laryngoscopies may be attempted by the same practitioner; then, the practitioner should be replaced and is permitted only 1 (max 2) attempt, as further instrumentation may lead to airway damage and even harder intubation conditions. If intubation is considered impossible after Plan A, the practitioner should

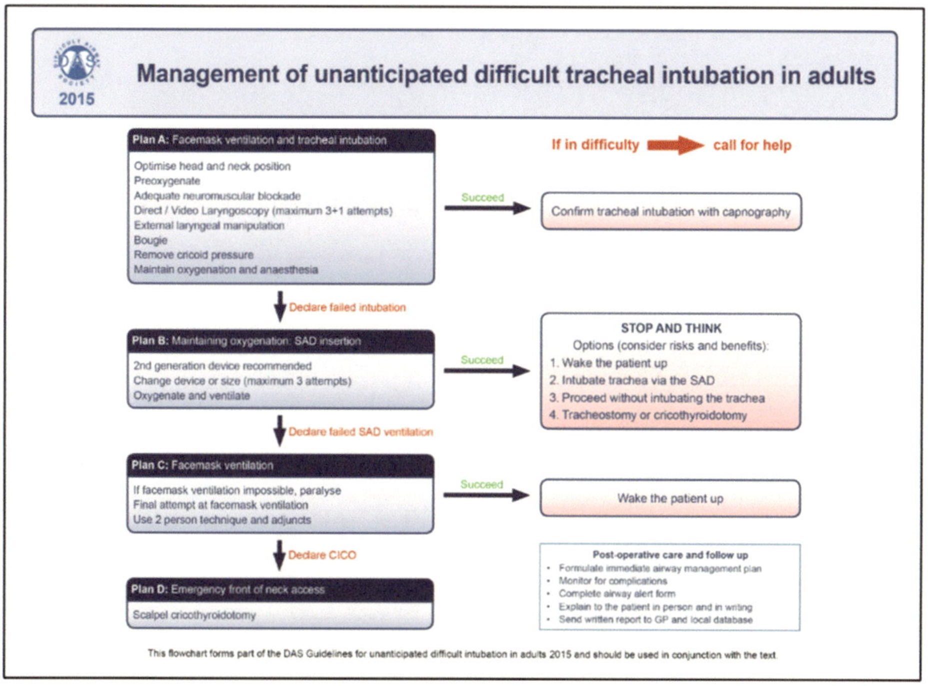

Figure 5.
Reproduced from "Difficult Airway Society 2015 guidelines for management of unanticipated difficult intubation in adults" C. Frerk, V. S. Mitchell, A. F. McNarry, C. Mendonca, R. Bhagrath, A. Patel, E. P. O'Sullivan, N. M. Woodall, and I. Ahmad, Difficult Airway Society.

proceed to Plan B and use the supraglottic device. In case of successful Plan B, the patient may be left with SAD, or the trachea may be intubated through the SAD. ILMA and ILA are most commonly used intubating suraglottic devices and are discussed above. There is still another method allowing ETT placement into trachea through SAD. A modified Bailey's maneuver may also be employed. The manipulation is described by incorporation of fiberoptic FASTRACH or Air-Q and then sliding the ETT (or ETT exchanger tube) into trachea under direct glottis visualization.

If Plan B has also failed, the patient should be started on ventilation again and woken up. If BMV is also unsuccessful, then switch to Plan C and perform immediate cricothyrotomy without delay.

7. Difficult airway management in special cases

- Obese patients are prone to airway wall collapse that restricts BMV. Any obese patient should be suspected to have difficult ventilation and difficult intubation. It is recommended to have a ready-to-use videolaryngoscope and employ it after the first unsuccessful intubation attempt. Do not forget that ramped head position (achieved by raising the patient's head with multiple pillows, to bring the external ear meatus on the same line with the sternum) alleviates laryngoscopy. At the other end, increased abdominal pressure and reduced lung reserve volume prone the patient to quick desaturation and high risk of aspiration. It is advantageous to ventilate the patient in Trendelenburg position, both to avoid aspiration

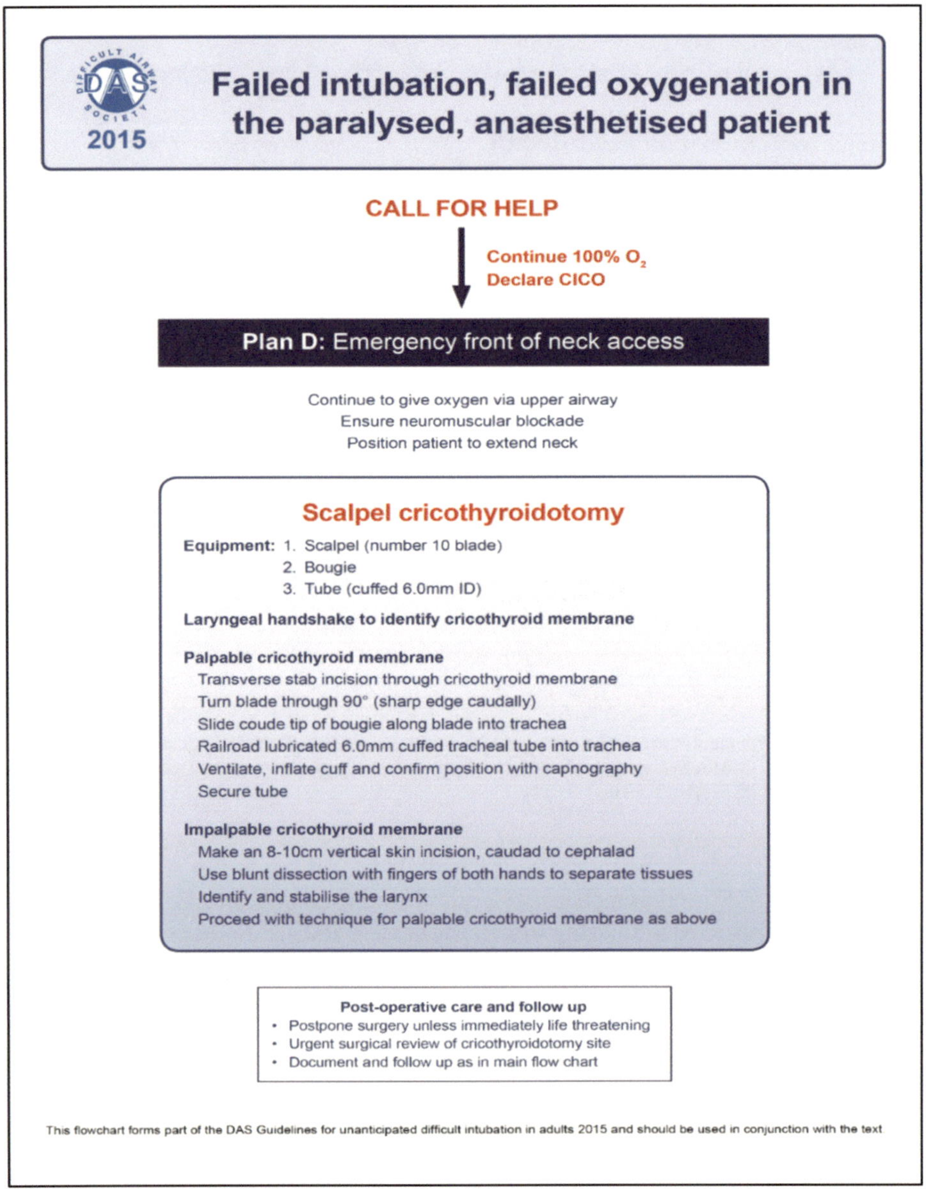

Figure 6.
Reproduced from "Difficult Airway Society 2015 guidelines for management of unanticipated difficult intubation in adults" C. Frerk, V. S. Mitchell, A. F. McNarry, C. Mendonca, R. Bhagrath, A. Patel, E. P. O'Sullivan, N. M. Woodall, and I. Ahmad, Difficult Airway Society.

and to sustain effective preoxygenation. Obese individuals pose difficulty at cricothyrotomy too. Due to excessive front neck fat tissue, identification of cricothyroid membrane is harder. Besides, the cricothyrotomy tube is usually too short to be advanced into the trachea, so scalpel—bougie technique and ETT insertion are preferred.

- Blunt or penetrating head and neck traumas, as well as blunt and penetrating direct airway traumas, burns are serious life threating conditions with concomitant difficult airway status. Neck fractures restrict cervical mobility and acute bleeding harden laryngoscopy; presence of burns leads to tissue swelling, and hematomas provide extra obstruction, all of which complicate airway device insertion. In such cases, it is of vital importance to diagnose if the airway obstruction is impending and manage airway protection before total failure occurs. In cases with visible tracheal laceration, take precautions to prevent tracheal retraction into airway. For this purpose, the trachea may be grasped with a clamp and immediate front-of-neck tracheotomy, and ETT placement should be performed. If there is no visible laceration of trachea, the practitioner should diagnose if the obstruction of airway is above or beneath the larynx. For cases with up-to-larynx obstruction and damage, steps for front-of-neck techniques are the only options. For cases with down-the-larynx obstruction or damage 'double setup' (simultaneous preparation for oral intubation and cricothyrotomy) or, even, 'triple setup' (simultaneous preparation for oral intubation, nonsurgical rescue device, and cricothyrotomy).

- Angioedema is another common difficult airway scenario faced in emergency departments. The goal is to evaluate how far the patient's airway is swelled. When diagnosing the patient, pay attention to uvula involvement. Asking the patient to pronounce his/her name may provide a concept about vocal cord involvement. İf both uvula and vocal cords are suspected to be swelled, awake fiberoptic intubation is the approach of choice. The chance for direct laryngoscope or videolaryngoscope intubation is extremely low. İf the patient admits with respiratory arrest, front-of-neck approach (may be combined with laryngoscopy attempt) should be undertaken immediately.

8. Conclusion

Although this chapter aimed to cover every single detail concerning difficult airway and its management, we still must mention that the final decision and approach is the practitioner's decision. İn reality, the practitioners face very complicated situations and usually are obligated to manage combination of difficult airway contexts, so the outcome is greatly influenced by the experience of the healthcare professional at the injured one's head.

Abbreviations

ASA	American Society of Anesthesiology
BMV	Bag mask ventilation
BURP	Backward-upward-rightward-pressure
CICO	Cannot intubate cannot oxygenate
CL	Cormack-Lehane
DA	Difficult airway
DAS	Difficult Airway Society
DSE	Skin-to-epiglottis distance
DSH	Skin-to-hyoid distance
DST	Skin-to-thyrohyoid membrane distance
ETT	Endotracheal tube

FBO	Fiberoptic
ILA	İntubating laryngeal airway
ILMA	İntubating laryngeal mask device
King LT	King laryngeal tube
LMA	Laryngeal mask airway
RAD	Retroglottic airway device
SAD	Supraglottic airway device
ULBT	Upper lip bite test
US	Ultrasound
USG	Ultrasound guidance

Author details

Nigar Kangarli* and Asım Esen
Bezmialem Vakif University, Istanbul, Türkiye

*Address all correspondence to: nikangarli@gmail.com

References

[1] Wong E, Ng YY. The difficult airway in the emergency department. International Journal of Emergency Medicine. 2008;**1**(2):107-111. DOI: 10.1007/s12245-008-003

[2] Pérez-Civantos D, Muñoz-Cantero A, Fuentes Morillas F, Nieto Sánchez P, Ángeles Santiago Triviño M, Durán CN. Management of new special devices for intubation in difficult airway situations [internet]. In: Special Considerations in Human Airway Management. London, UK: Intechopen; 2021. DOI: 10.5772/intechopen.97400

[3] Apfelbaum JL, Hagberg CA, Connis RT, Abdelmalak BB, Agarkar M, Dutton RP, et al. 2022 American Society of Anesthesiologists Practice Guidelines for management of the difficult airway. Anesthesiology. 2022;**136**:31-81. DOI: 10.1097/ALN.0000000000004002

[4] Antonakopoulos N, Bhide A. Focus on prenatal detection of micrognathia. Journal of Fetal Medicine. 2019;**6**:107-112

[5] Micrognathia—The Fetal Medicine Foundation [Internet]. [cited: February 26, 2021].

[6] Kaufman MG, Cassady CI, Hyman CH, Lee W, Watcha MF, Hippard HK, et al. Prenatal identification of Pierre Robin sequence: A review of the literature and look towards the future. Fetal Diagnosis and Therapy. 2016;**39**:81-89. DOI: 10.1159/000380948

[7] Faramarzi E, Soleimanpour H, Khan ZH, Mahmoodpoor A, Sanaie S. Upper lip bite test for prediction of difficult airway: A systematic review. Pakistan Journal of Medical Sciences. 2018;**34**(4):1019-1023. DOI: 10.12669/pjms.344.15364

[8] Dawood A, Talib B, Sabri I. Prediction of difficult intubation by using upper lip bite, thyromental distance and Mallampati score in comparison to Cormack and Lehane classification system. Wiadomości Lekarskie. 2021;**74**:2305-2314. DOI: 10.36740/wlek202109211

[9] Reed MJ et al. Can an airway assessment score predict difficulty at intubation in the emergency department? Emergency Medicine Journal. 2005;**22**:99-102

[10] Crosby ET, Cooper RM, Douglas MJ, Doyle DJ, Hung OR, Labrecque P, et al. The unanticipated difficult airway with recommendations for management. Canadian Journal of Anaesthesia. 1998;**45**:757-776

[11] Levitan RM, Everett WW, Ochroch EA. Limitations of difficult airway prediction in patients intubated in the emergency department. Annals of Emergency Medicine. 2004;**44**:307-313

[12] Ni H, Guan C, He G, et al. Ultrasound measurement of laryngeal structures in the parasagittal plane for the prediction of difficult laryngoscopies in Chinese adults. BMC Anesthesiology. 2020;**20**:134. DOI: 10.1186/s12871-020-01053-3

[13] Pinto J, Cordeiro L, Pereira C, Gama R, Fernandes HL, Assuncao J. Predicting difficult laryngoscopy using ultrasound measurement of distance from skin to epiglottis. Journal of Critical Care. 2016;**33**:26-31

[14] Falcetta S, Cavallo S, Gabbanelli V, Pelaia P, Sorbello M, Zdravkovic I, et al. Evaluation of two neck ultrasound measurements as predictors of difficult

direct laryngoscopy: A prospective observational study. European Journal of Anaesthesiology. 2018;**35**:1-8

[15] Chhabra AR, Thannappan S, Iyer HR. Preoperative ultrasonographic evaluation of the airway vis-à-vis the bedside airway assessment to predict potentially difficult airway on direct laryngoscopy in adult patients—A prospective, observational study. Ain-Shams Journal of Anesthesiology. 2023;**15**:2. DOI: 10.1186/s42077-022-00297-0

[16] Wu J, Dong J, Ding Y, Zheng J. Role of anterior neck soft tissue quantifications by ultrasound in predicting difficult laryngoscopy. Medical Science Monitor. 2014;**20**:2343-2350. DOI: 10.12659/MSM.891037

[17] Andruszkiewicz P, Wojtczak J, Sobczyk D, Stach O, Kowalik I. Effectiveness and validity of sonographic upper airway evaluation to predict difficult laryngoscopy. Journal of Ultrasound in Medicine. 2016;**35**:2243-2252. DOI: 10.7863/ultra.15.11098

[18] Nickson CH. Direct versus video laryngoscopy. In: Life in the Fast Lane. 2020.

[19] Li T, Jafari D, Meyer C, Voroba A, Haddad G, Abecassis S, et al. Video laryngoscopy is associated with improved first-pass intubation success compared with direct laryngoscopy in emergency department trauma patients. Journal of the American College of Emergency Physicians Open. 2021;**2**(1):e12373

[20] Sanchez A, Iyer RR, Morrison DE. Preparation of the patient for awake intubation. In: Hagberg CA, editor. Benumof's Airway Management: Principles and Practice. Philadelphia: Mosby-Elsevier; 2007. pp. 255-280

[21] Frerk C, Mitchell VS, McNarry AF, Mendonca C, Bhagrath R, Patel A, O'Sullivan EP, Woodall NM and Ahmad I. Difficult Airway Society 2015 Guidelines for Management of Unanticipated Difficult Intubation in Adults. Difficult Airway Society

Chapter 4

Airway Disorders as Predictive Factors of Exacerbations in Asthma and COPD

Hiroaki Kume, Natsumi Watanabe and Yasuhito Suzuki

Abstract

Asthma and chronic obstructive pulmonary disease (COPD) are heterogenous diseases in the respiratory system. Since wheezing, reduced FEV_1, eosinophilic airway inflammation, and airway hyperresponsiveness are observed in some patients with COPD similar to asthma, differential diagnosis is sometimes difficult in subset of these diseases. To advance the management and treatment of asthma and COPD, it is necessary to accurately classify patients with these two diseases according to distinct clinical phenotypes based on clinically meaningful outcomes such as symptoms, exacerbations, response to therapy, and prognosis. However, since several phenotypes are present in individual patients, a search for treatable traits needs to establish precision medicine for asthma and COPD. Since these diseases worsen with each repeated exacerbation, the establishment of treatment to avoid exacerbations is the most important goal of the long-term management of these diseases. Airway physiological and pathological disorders, such as reversibility in FEV_1, airway hyperresponsiveness, airway eosinophilic inflammation, and upper respiratory infection, are probably considered as major predictors of exacerbations. This chapter states clinical phenotypes related to acute exacerbation to establish treatable traits for asthma and COPD.

Keywords: airway eosinophilia, airway hyperresponsiveness, lung function, phenotypes, treatable traits, precision medicine

1. Introduction

Not only bronchial asthma (asthma) but also chronic obstructive pulmonary disease (COPD) is generally considered as a common, preventable, and treatable disease, and these two diseases are complex and heterogeneous [1, 2]. Moreover, the differential diagnosis between elderly asthma and COPD is sometimes difficult using symptoms and lung function tests [3]. To indicate the complexity and heterogeneity concerning asthma and COPD, each patient with these two diseases should be meaningfully divided into groups according to similar clinical characteristics (clinical phenotypes). However, it has not been yet clinically established to identify and classify patients with these two diseases into defined subtypes according to distinct phenotypes. In these heterogenous diseases, individual patients can be stratified according to clinical phenotypes [4, 5]. Stratified medicine for these diseases based on distinct phenotypes is essential to advance toward personalize (precision) medicine, which is optimal medicine for these heterogenous and incurable diseases, such as asthma and COPD [6–8].

In recent years, longitudinal cohort studies for asthma [9] and COPD [10] were conducted to recognize the heterogeneity of these diseases. These cohort studies are probably beneficial to research clinical phenotypes, which are multiple characteristics in each disease, and for the development of treatable traits based on these distinct phenotypes, leading to the establishment of precision medicine in these two diseases. Each patient with these diseases can be grouped according to phenotypes, and these groupings are proposed to determine clusters of patients with common characteristics that relate to clinically meaningful outcomes such as symptoms, exacerbations, response to therapy, and prognosis (stratified medicine) [5, 11]. Furthermore, multifocal approaches to deal with diseases probably provide relevant information that can classify different subtypes of these diseases. Hence, these heterogeneous diseases should be assessed using multiple dimensions including clinical, physiological, imaging, and endotyping [8, 12].

Since severe exacerbations are closely related to comorbidity, prevention of acute exacerbations is a primary goal of management and therapy for asthma and COPD. Symptoms of these diseases possibly become worse based on various factors including upper airway infections, airway inflammation, comorbidities, and environmental risks [13]. In exacerbations, these two diseases have similar symptoms such as dyspnea, wheezing, chest tightness due to airway obstruction, and mucus production due to airway inflammation. Despite the present guideline-compliant therapy, acute exacerbations are not completely prevented in some cases of these diseases. Mild–moderate exacerbations require additional treatment such as rapid-acting bronchodilators, corticosteroids, and antibiotics. Repeated exacerbations result in a significant deterioration of lung function through airway remodeling [13, 14]. Accelerated loss of lung function in turn brings about increased risk of recurrent exacerbations in these patients, referred to as a vicious cycle. This phenomenon may cause the exacerbation-prone subset of asthma and COPD as novel phenotypes of these diseases [14, 15]. Functional and morphological alterations in the airways probably are associated with exacerbation triggers in these diseases.

Patients who are prone to exacerbations of asthma and COPD will deteriorate quality of life because of emergency visits and hospitalizations. Therefore, to stabilize symptoms related to these diseases in the future, it is necessary to search for distinct predictors of exacerbations. Moreover, it is desirable that suitable therapy for long-term management for these diseases should be established based on accurately predictable factors for exacerbations as treatable traits [14, 16–20]. This chapter states clinical phenotypes related to acute exacerbation to establish treatable traits for asthma and COPD.

2. Asthma

2.1 Clinical features

Although asthma is a common disease, diagnosis criteria are not clearly stated in the latest Global Initiative for Asthma (GINA) report [21]. Asthma is a heterogeneous and chronic respiratory disease, and airway inflammation and airway hyperresponsiveness are fundamentally pathophysiological features of this disease. These characteristics are beneficial to diagnose asthma accurately but are not clinically used much because the related methods of examinations such as sputum induction and methacholine provocation test are complicated. These characteristics are usually persisted even when symptoms are absent, and lung function is within normal limit. Moreover, it is quite difficult to return airway hyperresponsiveness to normal using conventional treatment with corticosteroids. However, the latest GINA report states that these two characteristics are not necessary and sufficient for the diagnosis of asthma [21], although they are probably therapeutic targets for the cure of asthma. This disease is generally diagnosed based on the history of respiratory symptoms (wheezing, dyspnea, chest tightness, and cough) that vary in intensity over time with variable expiratory airflow limitation (a reduction in forced expiratory volume in 1 second: FEV_1). These variations are often triggered by factors such as allergen exposure, exercise, and viral airway infections. The reversibility of airflow limitation is useful for the diagnosis of this disease, but this examination is probably low diagnostic sensitivity to asthma. The reversibility of airflow limitation is sometimes undetectable because lung function remains normal in many patients with asthma during a stable period.

2.2 Clinical phenotypes

Asthma is grouped as phenotype classifications according to their relative expression of symptoms and inflammation in primary care with predominantly mild to moderate disease and in secondary care with refractory disease populations [4]. Two groups, "early onset atopic" and "obese, noneosinophilic" is common and concordant in both care populations. In contrast, marked discordance is observed in secondary-care asthma between clusters "early onset symptom predominant" and "late-onset inflammation predominant", which is specific to refractory asthma [4]. The reasons for this dissociation are unclear; however, measurement of airway inflammation in these subgroups is probably beneficial to a reduction in exacerbation frequency in the inflammation-predominant group [4]. In another trial, distinct clinical phenotypes of severe asthma are classified into five categories using unsupervised hierarchical cluster analysis [22]: (1) early onset atopic asthma with normal lung function, (2) early onset atopic asthma with preserved lung function but increased medication requirements, (3) older obese women with late-onset nonatopic asthma, and (4, 5) severe airflow obstruction (Cluster 4: %FEV1 more than and equal to 65, Cluster 5: %FEV1 less than 65) [22]. Recently, cluster analysis for patients with asthma has been carried out based on a novel multidimensional approach, such as Th2, non-Th2, and mixed inflammation in the natural history of asthma [23, 24]. The risk factors (genetic variants and environmental exposures) and the molecular mechanisms (endotypes) may interact in complex manners in each patient, and they are shared by some, but not all, patients [20]. The latest GINA report states that phenotypes of asthma similarly are identified in five clusters according to clinical and pathophysiological features, that is, (1) allergic, (2) nonallergic, (3) adult-onset, (4) persistent airflow limitation, and (5) obesity [21]. However, except in patients with severe asthma, relationships are not clearly observed between the pathological characteristics and the clinical patterns or response to treatment. More studies are needed to establish the clinical utilities of phenotype classification in asthma [21].

2.3 Exacerbations

Patients with exacerbation-prone asthma generally have reduced lung function, such as forced expiratory volume in one second (FEV_1)/forced volume capacity (FVC), percent predicted FEV_1, percent predicted FVC, compared with other patients with asthma [25]. Exacerbations are generally considered to make symptoms and lung function worse than the usual condition. Although there is no clear consensus concerning asthma exacerbations, a severe exacerbation is defined as the need for treatment with systemic corticosteroids, emergency visits, and hospital admissions [26]. Environmental (respiratory virus, allergen, etc.) and personal factors (IgE, eosinophils, etc.) are associated with worsening symptoms and lung function in asthma [27]. Exacerbations are mostly triggered by viral infections in the upper airway; and airway eosinophilic inflammation induced by Th_2 cytokines is also generally considered to enhance susceptibility to exacerbations [28]. Moreover, another report has also indicated that regulation of Th_2 cytokine acts as phenotype/endotype-specific therapeutic targets for severe asthma management [29]. However, asthma exacerbations caused by low Th_2 phenotypes are difficult to distinguish physiologically and symptomatically from those caused by high Th_2 phenotypes [30]. It needs to be further understood concerning low Th_2 phenotypes. Major predictors associated with respiratory disorders for asthma exacerbations are shown in **Figure 1**.

2.3.1 Infection

Rhinoviruses mostly cause asthma exacerbations in children and adults. Infections of upper airway epithelial cells with Rhinovirus cause the release of pro-inflammatory cytokines and chemokines and the recruitment of inflammatory cells, such as neutrophils, lymphocytes, and eosinophils. Rhinovirus types are classified into three

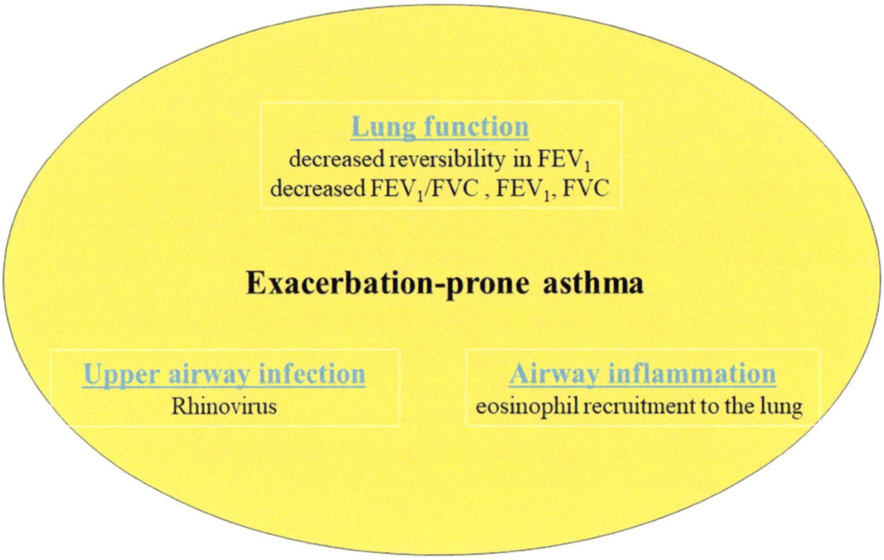

Figure 1.
Major predictors of exacerbations associated with respiratory disorders include function, infection, and inflammation in exacerbation-prone asthma. Illustrated based on Refs. [13, 25, 31, 32].

species (Rhinovirus-A, -B, and -C). Rhinovirus-A and -C are more likely to cause asthma exacerbations, and Rhinovirus-C infections in the upper airways are probably associated with severe asthma exacerbations and admission to intensive care for respiratory compromise [13]. In contrast, bacterial infections may not be so closely related to acute asthma exacerbations. However, respiratory virus infections in the upper airways may impair the antibacterial defenses, resulting in emergence of bacterial infections or changes in the microbiome.

2.3.2 Reversibility of airflow limitation

Reversibility of airway obstruction (airflow limitation) is proven by an increase of FEV_1 of more than 12% and 200 mL from baseline after inhalation of a short-acting β_2-adrenergic agonist using spirometry, and this bronchodilator reversibility is considered not only a recommended diagnostic criteria for asthma but also an indicator of stable long-term management of this disease. The maximal post-bronchodilator reversibility is associated with the frequency of asthma exacerbations [13, 25]. In contrast, other clinical reports have indicated that reversibility of airflow limitation is not always associated with asthma exacerbations [33], and that reduced bronchodilator reversibility is a risk factor against sensitivity to asthma therapy and is related to future asthma exacerbations [34]. It remains controversial whether the reversibility of airflow limitation can be a predictive factor for asthma exacerbations. A lack of reversibility in airflow limitation may be observed in a deterioration of lung function (airway remodeling) due to poor long-term management; in contrast, this phenomenon is also observed in an amelioration of lung function due to good long-term management. Therefore, the reversibility of airflow limitation may be insufficient to accurately evaluate long-term asthma management status.

2.3.3 Airway hyperresponsiveness

Airway hyperresponsiveness is a fundamental feature in the pathophysiology of asthma. This characteristic pathophysiology is represented as increased reactivity to muscarinic receptor agonists (acetylcholine and methacholine), histamine, and mannitol in the airway. The inhalation provocation test using these contractile agonists is clinically performed to examine airway hyperresponsiveness, which is diagnosed as threshold values of 8 mg/mL in these agents when the cumulative dose curve causing a 20% reduction in FEV_1 (PC_{20}) was calculated in the inhalation challenge test using these agents [35, 36]. However, the latest GINA report states that airway hyperresponsiveness is not necessary to make the diagnosis of asthma [21]. Since airway hyperresponsiveness is resistant to the currently recommended treatment using inhaled corticosteroids, it is generally considered that asthma cannot be cured. The severity of airway hyperresponsiveness may related to instability of symptoms or frequency of exacerbations. However, the relationship between asthma exacerbations and airway hyperresponsiveness still remains unclear. Although the inhalation provocation test using these contractile agents has the highest sensitivity to diagnose asthma, this provocation test to detect airway hyperresponsiveness is not always performed routinely for clinical diagnosis of asthma, probably because of its complexity. A recent clinical study has demonstrated that tezepelumab, a human anti-thymic stromal lymphopoietin (TSLP) monoclonal antibody, may reduce airway hyperresponsiveness to mannitol in patients with refractory asthma [37]. In vitro studies have shown that hyperresponsiveness to muscarinic agonists (airway hyperresponsiveness) is inhibited through the inactivation of Rho-kinase, a target molecule of RhoA (a monomeric GTP-binding protein) in airway smooth muscle [38, 39]. Since Rho-kinase, an inhibitor of myosin phosphatase, contributes to contraction, cell migration, cell proliferation, and reorganization of actin cytoskeleton through Ca^{2+} sensitization, this molecule is probably a therapeutic target for airflow limitation, airway hyperresponsiveness, eosinophil recruitment, and airway remodeling, which are the major features of asthma [40, 41].

2.3.4 Airway eosinophilia

Eosinophilic airway inflammation (eosinophil recruitment to the airways) is also a fundamental feature in the pathophysiology of asthma. However, the latest GINA report also states that airway eosinophilia is not necessary or sufficient to make the diagnosis of asthma [21]. Allergen challenges cause eosinophil recruitment to the airways in a sensitized mouse model of asthma, and this phenomenon is attenuated in the presence of Rho-kinase inhibitors [39]. Eosinophil recruitment to the airways is also clinically observed not only in unstable asthma [31] but also in stable asthma [42]. Eosinophilic airway inflammation is probably associated with symptoms and exacerbations in unstable periods in asthma, but little is unknown about the meaning of eosinophilic airway inflammation in stable periods in this disease. In pathological findings using bronchoscope, eosinophil infiltration to the distal airways is associated with nocturnal symptoms in patients with asthma [31]. Small airway eosinophilia may be involved in asthma exacerbations [43]. However, since clinical examination for small airways has not been established yet, details are unknown about it. Although sputum examination is a minimally invasive and accurate method to evaluate airway inflammation, the cut-off value (a criterion value for clinical diagnosis) is not established yet in quantitative analysis of sputum examination, but eosinophilic airway inflammation is generally defined as eosinophil fraction more than 3% [32]. In contrast, blood tests and fractional exhaled nitric oxide (FeNO) are clinically used widely, probably because of their convenience, but these values may be inaccurate because of indirect measurements for airway inflammation. A previous clinical trial has demonstrated that a treatment strategy due to normalization of sputum eosinophil count markedly reduces asthma exacerbations and admissions with the need for additional anti-asthma agents, compared with a standard management strategy due to guidelines [32]. Among four measures of Th_2-related inflammation (eosinophil counts in blood and sputum, FeNO, IgE), a reduction in the sputum eosinophils markedly suppresses the frequency of asthma exacerbations; in contrast, other three clinical examinations related to Th_2 inflammation are not associated with a reduction in asthma exacerbations [26]. Therefore, the number of eosinophils in the sputum examination is probably a predictor for asthma exacerbations as a future risk.

3. COPD

3.1 Clinical features

Chronic obstructive lung disease (COPD) is also generally considered a heterogenous, preventable, and treatable disease that is defined as persistent respiratory symptoms (shortness of breath, chronic cough, and sputum production) and persistent airway obstruction (airflow limitation) that will not return to the normal range [44]. The pathogenesis of COPD is brought about by chronic lung inflammation due to oxidative stress through cigarette smoke and other environmental exposures (biomass fuel, air pollution, etc.) [45]. Responses to chronic lung inflammation caused by neutrophils and macrophages are modified in patients with COPD, leading to emphysema and small airway fibrosis (the pathological features of this disease). Since COPD is diagnosed only based on persistent airflow limitation in spirometry, but because FEV_1/FVC physiologically decreases with age, the fixed cut-off point for FEV_1/FVC ratio < 70% may be inaccurate to use for diagnosis of COPD may result in overdiagnosis of COPD in older adults. The airflow limitation is progressive, and a decline of FEV_1 varies in each patient with COPD. The loss of alveolar attachment to the small airways causes not only airflow limitation but also gas trapping, such as an increase in residual volume (RV) or a decrease in inspiratory capacity (IC), other than airflow limitation due to the loss of alveolar attachment to the small airways. Since COPD is associated with small airway and alveolar damage [46], some cases of COPD develop a low lung diffusing capacity for carbon monoxide (DL_{CO}). A reduction in FEV_1 is not always related to shortness of breath in patients with COPD; in contrast, a reduction in IC and an increase in RV cause shortness of breath through dynamic hyperinflation. Moreover, abnormities of DLco probably cause shortness of breath through hypoxemia via a reduction in diffusion capacity during exercise. It is generally considered that airflow limitation could be observed in a variety of overlapping conditions among airway inflammatory diseases in patients with COPD and asthma [47, 48]. Moreover, airway eosinophilia and airway hyperresponsiveness probably develop in a subset of COPD as clinical phenotypes similar to asthma [3].

3.2 Clinical phenotypes

As the first phenotype classification, COPD was separated into two groups, such as the "Pink Puffers" and the "Blue Bloaters" [49]. However, COPD has complexity and heterogeneity in symptoms, progression, exacerbations, functional outcomes, and response to treatment, pathogenesis, and pathology [5, 50]. Hence, it is desirable to meaningfully identify and classify groups of patients with similar clinical characteristics, referred to as clinical phenotypes. However, it has not been established to classify patients with COPD into defined subtypes according to distinct phenotypes for clinical use. Patients with this disease should be stratified according to clinical phenotypes [5, 16, 51]. Stratified medicine is needed to assess multiple dimensions that include clinical (symptoms, exacerbations, and comorbidity), physiologic (airflow limitation, impaired diffusion, airway trapping, small airway dysfunction, and airway hyperresponsiveness), imaging (emphysema and small airway narrowing), and endotyping (inflammatory profiling) dimensions [5, 8, 11, 12], resulting in classifications of patients to distinct prognostic and therapeutic subgroups for both clinical and research purposes as a heterogeneous disease in COPD. However, clinical characteristics is mixed in various proportions in individual patients with COPD. Ever since 2011, the Global Initiative for Chronic Obstructive Lung Disease (GOLD) report states a multidimensional assessment of patients with COPD that includes two new dimensions: symptoms experienced by the patient and the risk of future exacerbations. Even though symptoms disappear through treatment for an exacerbation, the severity of COPD may not be decreased. Since COPD gradually worsens with each exacerbation, it is very important to know what characteristics patients prone to exacerbations have. A group of subjects with 2 or more exacerbations per year is considered as frequent exacerbator of COPD [14, 44]. Therefore, searches for phenotypes in COPD prone to exacerbations are beneficial to advance the management and treatment of COPD. Major predictors associated with respiratory disorders for COPD exacerbations are shown in **Figure 2**.

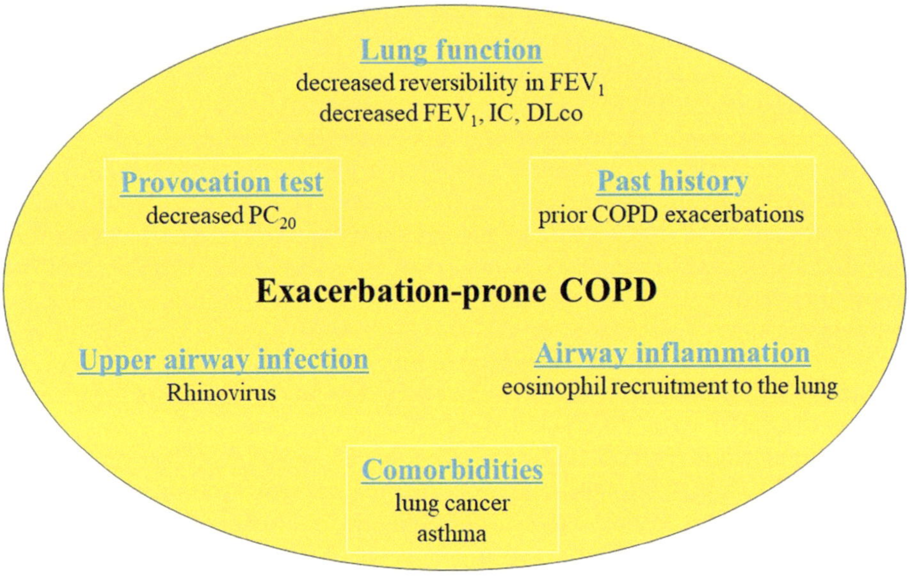

Figure 2.
In exacerbation-prone COPD, major predictors of exacerbations are associated with respiratory disorders such as function, hyperresponsiveness, infection, diseases, inflammation, and prior exacerbations. Illustrated based on Refs. [3, 14, 52–58].

3.3 Exacerbations

3.3.1 Prior exacerbations

A longitudinal trial enrolled 2138 patients with COPD has been performed to evaluate predictors of exacerbations over 3 years (the Evaluation of COPD Longitudinally to Identify Predictive Surrogate Endpoints: ECLIPSE study) [14]. Exacerbations were defined as additional treatments by antibiotics or corticosteroids and hospitalization (severe exacerbations). This clinical study has indicated that the most reliable predictor of exacerbations is a history of prior exacerbations, referred to as a frequent exacerbation phenotype [14]. Recently, another clinical study has been performed to evaluate the history of exacerbations and other factors as predictors over 1 year (the Acute COPD Exacerbation Prediction Tool: ACCEPT) [59]. Predicted and observed exacerbation rates in this study are similar to the results shown in the ECLIPSE study [59]. A literature review has indicated that exacerbation history within the past year is also a reliable predictor of future exacerbations [52], and there is a significant relationship between exacerbation history and risk of future moderate-to-severe exacerbations [52]. The late GOLD report states that COPD is classified into four stages (Grade I–IV) based on the percentage predicted FEV_1. Modified Medical Research Council (mMRC) Dyspnea Scale and exacerbation history are each divided into two to form four groups A–D [21]. This assessment approach will guide more precise treatment toward individualized patients with COPD. However, this classification is still insufficient to express the heterogeneity of COPD accurately.

3.3.2 Comorbidities

Many previous reports have indicated that comorbidities are associated with the occurrence of moderate-to-severe exacerbations [52]. Comorbidities related to moderate-to-severe exacerbations include various diseases (malignancy, cardiovascular, respiratory comorbidities, etc.) [52]. Among these comorbidities, cardiovascular diseases are most closely associated with COPD readmissions in the emergency room. The number of comorbidities also augments the degree of risk for both moderate and severe exacerbations. Chronic comorbidities frequently develop in COPD; 88% of patients with COPD have at least one comorbidity, such as hypertension, coronary heart disease, osteoarthritis, etc. [53]. Moreover, the comorbidities related to the great risk of frequent exacerbations are pulmonary cancer, heart failure, and asthma [53]. Since airway disorders (infection, airflow limitation, hyperresponsiveness) overlap in subset of asthma and COPD, asthma can be a predictor for COPD exacerbations.

3.3.3 Infections

When infections develop in patients with COPD, stable periods are sometimes interrupted by acute worsening of respiratory symptoms, and additional treatments are required (exacerbations). In acute COPD exacerbation periods, pathological microorganisms (bacteria, viruses) are observed in the lower airway secretions with a relatively high frequency [60]. *Hemophilus influenzae*, *Streptococcus pneumoniae*, and *Moraxella catarrhalis* are the most common bacterial pathogens for exacerbations [61]. However, viral infections in the upper respiratory system are more closely related to COPD exacerbations. Rhinovirus is most frequently associated with exacerbations [54], whereas Coronavirus, Parainfluenza, Adenovirus, and Influenza viruses are less prevalent. In addition to these acute infections, persistent chronic systemic inflammation can be attributed to the frequency of COPD exacerbations. When patients with COPD are divided into low and high interleukin 6 (IL-6) groups, more frequent exacerbations are observed in the high IL-6 group than in the low IL-6 group. The values of IL-6 (14.03 pg./mL or more) can be a predictor for two or more COPD exacerbations in the following year [62].

3.3.4 Lung function

COPD with a normal lung function in early adulthood is related to a higher risk of mortality than that with a reduced lung function already in early adulthood; however, the clinical relevance of the attained FEV_1 trajectory to exacerbations is still unknown in this report [63]. Many clinical trials have indicated that mean increases in trough FEV_1 cause significant decreases in exacerbations and hospitalizations [64], indicating that treatment effects on FEV1 can avoid the future risk of COPD. The annual decline in FEV_1 is related to the annual exacerbation rate but not to mortality [55]. Furthermore, a literature review has demonstrated that there is a positive relationship between the risk of future COPD exacerbations and lack of bronchodilator reversibility in FEV_1 [52] and that four stages of (Grade I–IV) based on the percentage predicted FEV_1 is not related to future COPD exacerbations [52]. Measurement of DLco was not carried out in some large cohort studies, such as ECLIPSE, but a previous clinical study with a relatively small sample size has suggested that a reduction in DLco is related to the frequency of COPD exacerbations [56]. In the meta-analysis, DL_{CO} % predicted is significantly lower in the high exacerbation risk group in the GOLD report (group C/D) than in the low exacerbation risk group in the GOLD report (group A/B); and DL_{CO} % predicted is also lower in frequent exacerbators than in nonexacerbators [65]. In analysis from the Genetic Epidemiology of COPD (COPDGene) study, a reduction in DL_{CO} of 10% predicted to cause approximately

14% higher rate of hospitalization for COPD exacerbations [57]. Moreover, impairments in DLco (50% predicted or less) are independently associated with an increased rate of severe exacerbations, and combined impairments in DLco and FEV_1 (both 50% predicted or less) further increase the rate of severe exacerbations [57]. A reduction in IC due to an increase in RV causes shortness of breath through hyperinflation independent of hypoxemia. A clinical trial has indicated that the IC percentage predicted is significantly reduced in COPD with frequent exacerbations, and the Motley index (RV/total lung capacity (TLC) percentage) is also significantly increased in these patients with COPD [58]. Therefore, FEV_1, DLco, IC, and RV/TLC can be predictors for COPD exacerbations.

3.3.5 Airway hyperresponsiveness

Airway hyperresponsiveness is conventionally considered a hallmark of asthma; however, it has been recently proven that this pathophysiological feature is also observed in approximately 45% of patients with COPD [3, 66]. Airway hyperresponsiveness in COPD is not related to eosinophil recruitment to the lung and complications of asthma [3]. The methods of the inhalation provocation test and diagnosis of airway hyperresponsiveness are described in Section 2.3.3. Since FEV_1 is markedly reduced in a subset of COPD, the inhalation provocation test should be performed in the limited cases with FEV_1 70% or more of predicted values to avoid the occurrence of risk of respiratory failure and the production of false positive results [3]. A recent clinical trial has demonstrated that COPD exacerbations occur much more frequently in patients who have airway hyperresponsiveness than in patients who do not have that, and airway hyperresponsiveness is considered a predictor for COPD exacerbations and can be a treatable trait for this disease, similar to asthma [3]. Although there is currently no treatment for airway hyperresponsiveness related to COPD, tezepelumab (human anti-TSLP monoclonal antibody) and Rho-kinase inhibitors may be effective for airway hyperresponsiveness related to COPD, similar to asthma, as described in Section 2.3.3. [38, 40].

3.3.6 Airway eosinophilia

Eosinophilic airway inflammation is conventionally considered the essential pathophysiology of asthma, as described in Section 2.3.4.; however, it has been recently proven that eosinophil recruitment to the lung (3% or more of sputum eosinophil) is also recognized in approximately 35% of patients with COPD independent of asthma using sputum induction [3, 67]. Airway eosinophilia should be evaluated using sputum eosinophil counts because blood eosinophil counts cannot directly reflect airway conditions and cannot accurately evaluate eosinophilic airway inflammation. Daily administration of inhaled corticosteroids is effective for these patients with COPD who have higher values of sputum eosinophil, and few exacerbations occurred in these cases after induction of the inhaled corticosteroid therapy [3]. On the other hand, daily inhalation of corticosteroid was not administered to patients with COPD who have less than 3% of sputum eosinophil because eosinophilic airway inflammation is considered inactive. As a result, COPD exacerbation occurred more frequently in the untreated patients with lower values of sputum eosinophil counts than in the treated patients with higher values of sputum eosinophil count [3]. Although values of cutoff in sputum eosinophil counts are not established yet, less than 3% of sputum eosinophil is probably meaningful to detect airway eosinophilia.

Moreover, inhaled corticosteroids should be administered daily to patients with COPD who have qualitatively eosinophils in the sputum. Therefore, eosinophilic airway inflammation is considered a predictor for COPD exacerbations and can be a treatable trait.

4. Conclusions

Impaired physiological function and enhanced inflammation in the airways worsen symptoms (dyspnea, wheezing, and chest tightness) and require additional therapy (systemic corticosteroids and antibiotics), leading to hospitalization in some cases of asthma and COPD. Impaired lung function (decreases in FEV_1, IC, and DLco), decreased bronchodilation in response to β_2-adrenergic agonists (reversibility in FEV_1), and increased bronchoconstriction in response to muscarinic agonists (airway hyperresponsiveness) are probably predictors of acute exacerbations for these diseases. Furthermore, eosinophil recruitment to the lung (airway eosinophilia) and viral infections in the upper airways are also probably predictors of acute exacerbations for these diseases. These airway disorders can be treatable traits as clinical phenotypes for exacerbations-prone asthma and COPD. Advances in therapy for asthma and COPD need a search for distinct treatable traits for the prevention of acute exacerbations based on these predictors.

Conflict of interest

Hiroaki Kume: none.
Natsumi Watanabe: none.
Yasuhito Suzuki: none.

Author details

Hiroaki Kume*, Natsumi Watanabe and Yasuhito Suzuki
Department of Infectious Diseases and Respiratory Medicine, Fukushima Medical University Aizu Medical Center, Tanisawa, Kawahigashi, Aizuwakamatsu City, Fukushima, Japan

*Address all correspondence to: h-kume@fmu.ac.jp

References

[1] Rennard SI. COPD heterogeneity: What this will mean in practice. Respiratory Care. 2011;**56**(8):1181-1187. DOI: 10.4187/respcare.01419

[2] Papi A,Brightling C, Pedersen SE, et al. Asthma. Lancet. 2018;**391**(10122):783-800. DOI: 10.1016/S0140-6736(17)33311-1

[3] Kume H, Hojo M, Hashimoto N. Eosinophil inflammation and Hyperresponsiveness in the airways as phenotypes of COPD, and usefulness of inhaled Glucocorticosteroids. Frontiers in Pharmacology. 2019;**10**:765. DOI: 10.3389/fphar.2019.00765

[4] Haldar P, Pavord ID, Shaw DE, et al. Cluster analysis and clinical asthma phenotypes. American Journal of Respiratory and Critical Care Medicine. 2008;**178**(3):218-224. DOI: 10.1164/rccm.200711-1754OC

[5] Han MK, Agusti A, Calverley PM, et al. Chronic obstructive pulmonary disease phenotypes: The future of COPD. American Journal of Respiratory and Critical Care Medicine. 2010;**182**:598-604. DOI: 10.1164/rccm.200912-1843CC

[6] Agustí A, Bafadhel M, Beasley R, et al. Precision medicine in airway diseases: Moving to clinical practice. The European Respiratory Journal. 2017;**50**(4):1701655. DOI: 10.1183/13993003.01655-2017

[7] Louis R, Bureau F, Desmet CJ. Advances toward precision medicine for asthma. Biochemical Pharmacology. 2020;**179**:114081. DOI: 10.1016/j.bcp.2020.114081

[8] Kume H, Yamada R, Sato Y. New perspectives in pharmacological therapy for COPD: Phenotype classification and corticosteroids with bronchodilators. In: Ong KC, editor. A Compendium of Chronic Obstructive Pulmonary Disease. London, UK: IntchOpen; 2022. pp. 71-94. DOI: 10.5772/intechopen.106949

[9] Lavoie ME, Meloche J, Boucher-Lafleur AM, et al. Longitudinal follow-up of the asthma status in a French-Canadian cohort. Scientific Reports. 2022;**12**(1):13789. DOI: 10.1038/s41598-022-17959-6

[10] Ragland MF, Strand M, Baraghoshi D, et al. 10-year follow-up of lung function, respiratory symptoms, and functional capacity in the COPDGene study. Annals of the American Thoracic Society. 2022;**19**(3):381-388. DOI: 10.1513/AnnalsATS.202007-873OC

[11] Agustí A. Phenotypes and disease characterization in chronic obstructive pulmonary disease. Toward the extinction of phenotypes? Annals of the American Thoracic Society. 2013;**10**(Suppl):S125-S130. DOI: 10.1513/AnnalsATS.201303-055AW

[12] Segal LN, Martinez FJ. Chronic obstructive pulmonary disease subpopulations and phenotyping. The Journal of Allergy and Clinical Immunology. 2018;**141**:961-1971. DOI: 10.1016/j.jaci.2018.02.035

[13] Denlinger LC, Heymann P, Lutter R, et al. Exacerbation-prone asthma. The Journal of Allergy and Clinical Immunology. In Practice. 2020;**8**(2):474-482. DOI: 10.1016/j.jaip.2019.11.009

[14] Hurst JR, Vestbo J, Anzueto A, et al. Evaluation of COPD longitudinally to identify predictive surrogate endpoints

(ECLIPSE) investigators. Susceptibility to exacerbation in chronic obstructive pulmonary disease. The New England Journal of Medicine. 2010;**363**(12):1128-1138. DOI: 10.1056/NEJMoa0909883

[15] Dougherty RH, Fahy JV. Acute exacerbations of asthma: Epidemiology, biology and the exacerbation-prone phenotype. Clinical and Experimental Allergy. 2009;**39**(2):193-202. DOI: 10.1111/j.1365-2222.2008.03157.x

[16] Agusti A, Bel E, Thomas M, et al. Treatable traits: Toward precision medicine of chronic airway diseases. The European Respiratory Journal. 2016;**47**(2):410-419. DOI: 10.1183/13993003.01359-2015

[17] Silkoff PE, Moore WC, Sterk PJ. Three major efforts to phenotype asthma: Severe asthma research program, asthma disease Endotyping for personalized therapeutics, and unbiased biomarkers for the prediction of respiratory disease outcome. Clinics in Chest Medicine. 2019;**40**(1):13-28. DOI: 10.1016/j.ccm.2018.10.016

[18] Kaur R, Chupp G. Phenotypes and endotypes of adult asthma: Moving toward precision medicine. The Journal of Allergy and Clinical Immunology. 2019;**144**(1):1-12. DOI: 10.1016/j.jaci.2019.05.031

[19] Mathioudakis AG, Janssens W, Sivapalan P, et al. Acute exacerbations of chronic obstructive pulmonary disease: in search of diagnostic biomarkers and treatable traits. Thorax. 2020;**75**(6):520-527. DOI: 10.1136/thoraxjnl-2019-214484

[20] Schoettler N, Strek ME. Recent advances in severe asthma: From phenotypes to personalized medicine. Chest. 2020;**157**(3):516-528. DOI: 10.1016/j.chest.2019.10.009

[21] Global Initiative for Asthma. Global Strategy for Asthma Management and Prevention 2023. Available from: www:ginasthma.org

[22] Moore WC, Meyers DA, Wenzel SE, et al. National Heart, Lung, and Blood Institute's severe asthma research program. Identification of asthma phenotypes using cluster analysis in the severe asthma research program. American Journal of Respiratory and Critical Care Medicine. 2010;**181**(4):315-323. DOI: 10.1164/rccm.200906-0896OC

[23] Miller RL, Grayson MH, Strothman K. Advances in asthma: New understandings of asthma's natural history, risk factors, underlying mechanisms, and clinical management. The Journal of Allergy and Clinical Immunology. 2021;**148**(6):1430-1441. DOI: 10.1016/j.jaci.2021.10.001

[24] Ricciardolo FLM, Guida G, Bertolini F, et al. Phenotype overlap in the natural history of asthma. European Respiratory Review. 2023;**32**(168):220201. DOI: 10.1183/16000617.0201-2022

[25] Denlinger LC, Phillips BR, Ramratnam S, et al. National Heart, Lung, and Blood Institute's severe asthma research Program-3 investigators. Inflammatory and comorbid features of patients with severe asthma and frequent exacerbations. American Journal of Respiratory and Critical Care Medicine. 2017;**195**(3):302-313. DOI: 10.1164/rccm.201602-0419OC

[26] O'Byrne PM, Barnes PJ, Rodriguez-Roisin R, et al. Low dose inhaled budesonide and formoterol in mild persistent asthma: The OPTIMA randomized trial. American Journal of Respiratory and Critical Care Medicine. 2001;**164**(8 Pt 1):1392-1397. DOI: 10.1164/ajrccm.164.8.2104102

[27] Castillo JR, Peters SP, Busse WW. Asthma exacerbations: Pathogenesis, prevention, and treatment. The Journal of Allergy and Clinical Immunology. In Practice. 2017;**5**(4):918-927. DOI: 10.1016/j.jaip.2017.05.001

[28] Peters MC, Mauger D, Ross KR, et al. Evidence for exacerbation-prone asthma and predictive biomarkers of exacerbation frequency. American Journal of Respiratory and Critical Care Medicine. 2020;**202**(7):973-982. DOI: 10.1164/rccm.201909-1813OC

[29] Pelaia C, Crimi C, Vatrella A, et al. Molecular targets for biological therapies of severe asthma. Frontiers in Immunology. 2020;**11**:603312. DOI: 10.3389/fimmu.2020.603312

[30] McDowell PJ, Busby J, Hanratty CE, et al. Exacerbation profile and risk factors in a Type-2-low enriched severe asthma cohort: A clinical trial to assess asthma exacerbation phenotypes. American Journal of Respiratory and Critical Care Medicine. 2022;**206**(5):545-553. DOI: 10.1164/rccm.202201-0129OC

[31] Kraft M, Djukanovic R, Wilson S, et al. Alveolar tissue inflammation in asthma. American Journal of Respiratory and Critical Care Medicine. 1996;**154**(5):1505-1510. DOI: 10.1164/ajrccm.154.5.8912772

[32] Green RH, Brightling CE, McKenna S, et al. Asthma exacerbations and sputum eosinophil counts: A randomised controlled trial. Lancet. 2002;**360**(9347):1715-1721. DOI: 10.1016/S0140-6736(02)11679-5

[33] Janson C, Malinovschi A, Amaral AFS, et al. Bronchodilator reversibility in asthma and COPD: Findings from three large population studies. The European Respiratory Journal. 2019;**54**(3):1900561. DOI: 10.1183/13993003.00561-2019

[34] Liu L, Zhang X, Zhang L, et al. Reduced bronchodilator reversibility correlates with non-type 2 high asthma and future exacerbations: A prospective cohort study. Respiratory Medicine. 2022;**200**:106924. DOI: 10.1016/j.rmed.2022.106924

[35] Hargreave FE, Ryan G, Thomson NC, et al. Bronchial responsiveness to histamine or methacholine in asthma: Measurement and clinical significance. The Journal of Allergy and Clinical Immunology. 1981;**68**(5):347-355. DOI: 10.1016/0091-6749(81)90132-9

[36] Makino S, Ikemori R, Fukuda T, et al. Clinical evaluation of standard method of acetylcholine inhalation test in bronchial asthma. Arerugī. 1984;**33**(3):167-175. DOI: 10.15036/arerugi.33.167

[37] Diver S, Khalfaoui L, Emson C, et al. CASCADE study investigators. Effect of tezepelumab on airway inflammatory cells, remodeling, and hyperresponsiveness in patients with moderate-to-severe uncontrolled asthma (CASCADE): A double-blind, randomised, placebo-controlled, phase 2 trial. The Lancet Respiratory Medicine. 2021;**9**(11):1299-1312. DOI: 10.1016/S2213-2600(21)00226-5

[38] Kume H, Takeda N, Oguma T, et al. Sphingosine 1-phosphate causes airway hyper-reactivity by rho-mediated myosin phosphatase inactivation. The Journal of Pharmacology and Experimental Therapeutics. 2007;**320**(2):766-773. DOI: 10.1124/jpet.106.110718

[39] Taki F, Kume H, Kobayashi T, et al. Effects of rho-kinase inactivation on eosinophilia and hyper-reactivity in murine airways by allergen challenges. Clinical and Experimental Allergy. 2007;**37**(4):599-607. DOI: 10.1111/j.1365-2222.2007.02693.x

[40] Kume H. RhoA/Rho-kinase as a therapeutic target in asthma. Current Medicinal Chemistry. 2008;**15**(27):2876-2885. DOI: 10.2174/092986708786242831

[41] Wu X, Verschut V, Woest ME, et al. Rho-kinase 1/2 inhibition prevents transforming growth factor-β-induced effects on pulmonary remodeling and repair. Frontiers in Pharmacology. 2021;**11**:609509. DOI: 10.3389/fphar.2020.609509. eCollection 2020

[42] Belda J, Giner J, Casan P, et al. Mild exacerbations and eosinophilic inflammation in patients with stable, well-controlled asthma after 1 year of follow-up. Chest. 2001;**119**(4):1011-1017. DOI: 10.1378/chest.119.4.1011

[43] Kraft M, Richardson M, Hallmark B, et al. ATLANTIS study group. The role of small airway dysfunction in asthma control and exacerbations: A longitudinal, observational analysis using data from the ATLANTIS study. Lancet. Respiratory Medicine. 2022;**10**(7):661-668. DOI: 10.1016/S2213-2600(21)00536-1

[44] Global Initiative for Chronic Obstructive Lung Disease. Global Strategy for the Diagnosis, Management and Prevention of Chronic Obstructive Pulmonary Disease 2023 Report. Available from: www.goldcopd.org

[45] Kume H, Yamada R, Sato Y, et al. Airway smooth muscle regulated by oxidative stress in COPD. Antioxidants. 2023;**12**(1):142. DOI: 10.3390/antiox12010142

[46] Hogg JC. Pathophysiology of airflow limitation in chronic obstructive pulmonary disease. Lancet. 2004;**364**(9435):709-721. DOI: 10.1016/S0140-6736(04)16900-6

[47] American Thoracic Society. Standards for diagnosis and care of patients with chronic obstructive lung disease. American Journal of Respiratory and Critical Care Medicine. 1995;**152**:S77-S121

[48] Gibson PG, McDonald VM. Asthma-COPD overlap 2015: Now we are six. Thorax. 2015;**70**(7):683-691. DOI: 10.1136/thoraxjnl-2014-206740

[49] Dornhorst AC. Respiratory insufficiency. Lancet. 1955;**268**:1185-1187

[50] Spurzem JR, Rennard SI. Pathogenesis of COPD. Seminars in Respiratory and Critical Care Medicine. 2005;**26**(2):142-153. DOI: 10.1055/s-2005-869535

[51] Agusti A. The path to personalised medicine in COPD. Thorax. 2014;**69**(9):857-864. DOI: 10.1136/thoraxjnl-2014-205507

[52] Hurst JR, Han MK, Singh B, et al. Prognostic risk factors for moderate-to-severe exacerbations in patients with chronic obstructive pulmonary disease: A systematic literature review. Respiratory Research. 2022;**23**(1):213. DOI: 10.1186/s12931-022-02123-5

[53] Westerik JA, Metting EI, van Boven JF, et al. Associations between chronic comorbidity and exacerbation risk in primary care patients with COPD. Respiratory Research. 2017;**18**(1):31. DOI: 10.1186/s12931-017-0512-2

[54] Seemungal T, Harper-Owen R, Bhowmik A, et al. Respiratory viruses, symptoms, and inflammatory markers in acute exacerbations and stable chronic obstructive pulmonary disease. American Journal of Respiratory and Critical Care Medicine. 2001;**164**:1618-1623. DOI: 10.1164/ajrccm.164.9.2105011

[55] Alter P, Lucke T, Watz H, et al. Cardiovascular predictors of mortality and exacerbations in patients with COPD. Scientific Reports. 2022;**12**(1):21882. DOI: 10.1038/s41598-022-25938-0

[56] Lee HY, Kim JW, Lee SH, et al. Lower diffusing capacity with chronic bronchitis predicts higher risk of acute exacerbation in chronic obstructive lung disease. Journal of Thoracic Disease. 2016;**8**(6):1274-1282. DOI: 10.21037/jtd.2016.04.66

[57] Balasubramanian A, MacIntyre NR, Henderson RJ, et al. Diffusing capacity of carbon monoxide in assessment of COPD. Chest. 2019;**156**(6):1111-1119. DOI: 10.1016/j.chest.2019.06.035

[58] Capozzolo A, Carratù P, Dragonieri S, et al. Clinical and functional lung parameters associated with frequent Exacerbator phenotype in subjects with severe COPD. Respiratory Care. 2017;**62**(5):572-578. DOI: 10.4187/respcare.05278

[59] Adibi A, Sin DD, Safari A, et al. The acute COPD exacerbation prediction tool (ACCEPT): A modelling study. The Lancet Respiratory Medicine. 2020;**8**(10):1013-1021. DOI: 10.1016/S2213-2600(19)30397-2

[60] Monsó E, Ruiz J, Rosell A, Manterola J, er al. Bacterial infection in chronic obstructive pulmonary disease. A study of stable and exacerbated outpatients using the protected specimen brush. American Journal of Respiratory and Critical Care Medicine. 1995;**152**:1316-1320. DOI: 10.1164/ajrccm.152.4.7551388

[61] Sethi S, Sethi R, Eschberger K, et al. Airway bacterial concentrations and exacerbations of chronic obstructive pulmonary disease. American Journal of Respiratory and Critical Care Medicine. 2007;**176**:356-361. DOI: 10.1164/rccm.200703-417OC

[62] Huang H, Huang X, Zeng K, et al. Interleukin-6 is a strong predictor of the frequency of COPD exacerbation within 1 year. International Journal of Chronic Obstructive Pulmonary Disease. 2021;**16**:2945-2951. DOI: 10.2147/COPD.S332505

[63] Marott JL, Ingebrigtsen TS, Çolak Y, et al. Lung function trajectories leading to chronic obstructive pulmonary disease as predictors of exacerbations and mortality. American Journal of Respiratory and Critical Care Medicine. 2020;**202**(2):210-218. DOI: 10.1164/rccm.201911-2115OC

[64] Martin AL, Marvel J, Fahrbach K, et al. The association of lung function and St. George's respiratory questionnaire with exacerbations in COPD: A systematic literature review and regression analysis. Respiratory Research. 2016;**17**:40. DOI: 10.1186/s12931-016-0356-1

[65] Ni Y, Yu Y, Dai R, et al. Diffusing capacity in chronic obstructive pulmonary disease assessment: A meta-analysis. Chronic Respiratory Disease. 2021;**18**:14799731211056340. DOI: 10.1177/14799731211056340

[66] Zanini A, Cherubino F, Zampogna E, et al. Bronchial hyperresponsiveness, airway inflammation, and reversibility in patients with chronic obstructive pulmonary disease. International Journal of Chronic Obstructive Pulmonary Disease. 2015;**10**:1155-1161. DOI: 10.2147/COPD.S80992

[67] Leigh R, Pizzichini MM, Morris MM, et al. Stable COPD: Predicting benefit from high-dose inhaled corticosteroid treatment. The European Respiratory Journal. 2006;**27**(5):964-971. DOI: 10.1183/09031936.06.00072105

Chapter 5

Awake Tracheal Intubation in the Emergency Department

Erick Dunkley-Pinnock

Abstract

Awake tracheal intubation is a valid and highly recommended option for any situation where significant anticipated difficult intubation is expected. Despite expert recommendations and available video assisted device it's not a common practice and it still underuse because it seems as a very complex procedure. With a well-structured protocol, education and training, most health care personnel in the emergency department could perform it in a matter of minute, without delaying urgent care and maintaining a patent airway for adequate oxygenation.

Keywords: awake, tracheal, intubation, video-assisted devices, emergency, guidelines

1. Introduction

1.1 Awake tracheal intubation definition

Awake tracheal intubation (ATI) is define as a technique where the patient is intubated without the need of sedative or paralytic agent, but instead with the use of local anesthetics the airway is numb to maintain an adequate ventilation and oxygenation [1, 2].

1.2 History and evolution throughout time

First described by Sir William MacEwen, a Scottish surgeon, in 1880 of a patient suffering from obstruction of a tumor from the base of the tongue [3]. Soon after in 1881, ATI under topical anesthesia with cocaine, was first describe by Franz Kuhn, a German surgeon. Since then, orotracheal intubation trough the mouth as suffered several modifications, from external, digital palpation of the pharynx and upper tracheal structure to the visualization of the vocal cords by direct laryngoscopy [4, 5]. In 1967 a year before the introduction of fiberoptic bronchoscopy (FOB) in clinical practice by Kensuke Ikeda of Japan, an English anesthetist, Peter Murphy used it to aid in the nasal intubation of a patient with Still's disease [6]. Since the 90's ATI with

FOB has been recognized as a standard of care by different airway society practice guideline for the management of difficult airway, reporting a success rate of 88 to 100% in anticipated difficult airway patients [7].

1.3 Indications and contraindications

It is the standard of care for the management of anticipated airway in many practice guidelines, and it is recommended anytime there is suspected difficult laryngoscopy or facemask ventilation [8]. But there are some specific pathologies that are common practice for patient requiring ATI in the emergency department and are not limited to morbid obesity with a body mass index (BMI) of 40 or higher, pathology of the head and neck (large tumor, angioedema, obstructive sleep apnea) and a history of difficult intubation in the past. The only valid contraindication is a patient not accepting the procedure or not able to cooperative because of nonresponsive or altered mental status.

1.4 Incidence and statistics (difficult intubation and awake tracheal intubation)

The incidence of ATI in the emergency department is low (0.4%) [9] and it is lower than the incidence of difficult laryngoscopy in trauma patient in the emergency (between 12 and 14%) [10]. Reports suggest lack of familiarity and experience are the most common reasons.

1.5 Implementation in the emergency room settings. Controversies and discussions

This cause underutilization in those emergency department where other techniques like rapid sequence intubation (RSI) are more common [11]. This in part because of a strong believe that patient will not accept the procedure if asked. A qualitative, descriptive study in Sweden demonstrate that most patient undergoing ATI when tailored information and breathing instruction are giving during the procedure would not hesitate to undergo awake intubation again in the future if needed. The information provided should not overwhelm the patient with details about technical issues, instead it should cover basic knowledge of a stepwise approach and anticipate expected event like the discomfort if the nasal route if selected or possible complication like bleeding and how can it be corrected [12].

1.6 Benefits of awake tracheal intubation

There are several benefits with ATI, mostly because it permit and secure a patent airway to avoid the risk of low blood oxygen (hypoxemia) or high blood carbon dioxide (hypercapnia) [11] or the risk of food aspiration in the bronchi because protective laryngeal reflexes are preserved [8], and also to avoid the risk associated with induction agent commonly use in RSI like low blood pressure (hypotension) and slow heart rate (bradycardia) that could impended hemodynamic stability and increase morbidity and mortality.

2. Preparation

2.1 Patient selection

Selecting the right patient for ATI is the most difficult part. There is no evidence that support any individual method developed specifically for ATI and overall difficult airway predictions methods are unreliable, making all intubations potentially difficult in the emergency room [2, 13]. Despite these steps back emergency doctor most perform in a timely manner an in-depth history, targeting past difficult airway problem and how there were managed, followed by a thorough examination of the airway.

2.2 Cognitive aids

The use of cognitive aid can accelerate this process and it is highly recommended by difficult airway international guidelines [2]. Checklist and visual maps can help on decision making in environment such as the emergency room, who needs a rapid response, team collaboration and assurance that those who participate have a specific set of tasks.

2.3 Clinical and physical evaluation

Sign and symptoms could help in the decision making when it comes to perform intubation in a conscious patient with neck tumor or mass [14]. Some of these could be and not limited to acute change in voice, history of difficult breathing (dyspnea), difficult swallowing (dysphagia) with or without salivation, dyspnea not tolerated when lying flat only in the seated position. A physical examination could reveal difficult airway parameter (e. g. a Mallampati scale III or IV), large front of neck mass or tracheal deviation by visualization or palpation.

2.4 Imaging analysis and labs test

In an environment like the emergency room imaging evaluation at the bedside could facilitate airway assessment and safe time without the need for transporting the patient to the MRI or CT scan room. Two techniques have demonstrated high sensitivity and specificity and can be used for decision making. These are ultrasound and transnasal endoscopy or nasopharyngoscopy [7, 15]. Ultrasound could help in the assessment of tracheal deviation or obstruction in the presence of large front of neck mass or tissue. Also, it has been used in the emergency room for visualization of the cricoid membrane for urgent cricoidectomy to maintain ventilation if needed [15].

Difficulty	Physical examination	Hemodynamics and comorbidities	Recommended position	Probable outcomes
Low	• Mallampati scale I • Mouth opening >3 cm. • Thyromental distance >6 cm • Normal neck range mobility • Small mass tumor • Tolerate decubitus position.	• O_2 saturation > 95% • No supplemental O_2 • Neurologic integrity intact • Stable cardiovascular system	• Lying down	• Mild or no complications
	• Mallampati scale II or III • Mouth opening < 3 cm. • Thyromental distance <6 cm. • Limited Neck mobility • Medium size mass (less than 50% occlusion).	• O_2 saturation 90–95% • Moderate supplemental O2 • Neurologic integrity intact • Stable cardiovascular system	• Semirecumbent position r or head up at a 30° angle	• Desaturation • Hypoxia • Gastric aspiration
High	• Mallampati scale IV • Mouth opening less than 3 cm. • Thyromental distance <5 cm • No neck mobility o used of neck immobilization. • Large neck mass (80% occlusion or more) • Salivation, stridor • Cannot tolerate decubitus. • BMI > 45 kg/m^2	• O2 saturation < 90% • Despite supplemental oxygen therapy. • Impaired Neurologic integrity: drowsiness, lethargic. • Unstable cardiovascular system (hypotension, bradycardic)	• Semirecumbent position or completely seated.	• Hypoxia • Hypercapnia • Bradycardia • Tachycardia • Hypertension • Hypotension • Heart failure • Death

Table 1.
Cognitive aid for decision making for the selection of patient when considering awake tracheal intubation.

Above (**Table 1**) we use several patient characteristics to help guide clinicians in the emergency room in decision making and patient selection in case of awake tracheal intubation if needed.

3. Equipment and materials

3.1 Video assisted devices

Fiberoptic intubation (FOI) has been the standard method for many years in the management of difficult airway and it is the mainstay in awake tracheal intubation, either nasally or orally [16]. The advancement of the technology as incorporated high quality video recording, increase the suction power and single use disposable devices which decrease the incidence of cross contamination, among others.

Videolaryngoscopy (VL) has gain in recent years more attention because it is more available, easier, and safer to use than FOI [8]. Familiarity has increased his use in non-operating room environment like the emergency area. The main limitations are with patient with limited mouth opening and large obstructive tumors that impairs visibility. The lack of a suction channel may cause difficulty in patient with increase secretion or blood making it impossible to visualize supraglottic structure. There is no evidence that show superiority over FOI [17].

Other devices like direct laryngoscopy and optical stylets have been used and evidence has not shown significant differences in time and success rate, therefore could also be considered as a valuable alternative [18]. One of the mayors causes in selecting one device over a another may be familiarity and availability [8, 17]. The use of cognitive aid like the table above (**Table 1**) could help in selecting the right equipment. For example, in cases where the risk is low the emergency physician could start with Videolaryngoscopy, direct laryngoscope or flexible stylet, when the difficulty increases, and the risk is high the main choice should be fully awake fiberoptic intubation in a seated position with a front of neck approach.

3.2 Setup/arrangement

Ergonomics study the interaction of the environment and its impact on performance and safety [2], when it comes to airway management in the emergency room, time constraints and lack of adequate space could make it challenging to meet adequate standard and performance. But still, we must maintain the same standard as in the operating room (sterile gloves and gown, facemask, and continuous vital sign monitoring) [7].

Several factors should be considered before starting the procedure and everyone who is participating should be notify, these include patient position (seated, semirecumbent or lying down), the route of tracheal intubation (oral or nasal), visualization device (FOI or VL) and type of tracheal tube (reinforce or standard) [2]. If intubation is in the seated position a front of neck approach is the optimal choice, with the operator and assistant facing the patient, video monitor, patient vital sign monitor must be separate and in an adequate visible site for continuous monitoring. If the patient could tolerate lying down or semirecumbent position the operating physician could stand at the head of the patient and the assistant, other health personnel, video monitor and vital sign monitor on the opposite side towards the patient extremities. This approach is helpful and can be perform by the assistant in case head tilt or sniffing position it's needed because of obstruction from oversedation or increase secretion. We discussed before which video assisted device is adequate base on patient characteristics and underlying pathology (see above). Tracheal tube size is normally selected base on patient age group (pediatric, adults) and internal diameter (ID) but in patient with sign of important obstruction a smaller size or ID than needed should be selected. Comparison of reinforce tube versus standard polyvinylchloride (PVC) tube as shown that the first have superior outcome in terms of ease of tracheal intubation, railroading (advancing the tracheal tube over the flexible bronchoscope) and decreasing laryngeal impingement [2].

3.3 Medications

The three main objectives of premedication are: (1) Airway preparation, (2) Aspiration prophylaxis, (3) Anxiolysis and sedation. Airway preparation can be accomplished by application of antisialagogues, which are medication that decrease secretion in the mouth, pharynx, and bronchi, the most used are the antimuscarinic, and they also facilitate local anesthetics absorption allowing better absorption conditions. Commonly used clinical practice are atropine, glycopyrrolate and scopolamine. **Table 2**, summarize dosing regimen and principal characteristics of antimuscarinic drugs [13, 19].

If planning on using the nasal route, risk of bleeding is high because of highly vascular nasal mucosa and nasopharynx. Therefore, must be prepared with vasoconstrictor nose spray such has Phenylephrine 0.5% and Oxymetazoline 0.05%, which are applied topically 15 min before the procedure [13, 19].

Airway preparation with local anesthetics is a crucial part and an essential skill that should be dominated by physicians in the emergency room. The most commonly use drugs are lidocaine (2%) and tetracaine (1%) solutions or prepared canned spray [20]. Local anesthetics can be applied via topical or nerve block techniques. Topical administration could be applied by several ways, direct application using solution-soaked sponge or gauze, spraying directly to the oropharynx, or nebulizing the entire airway mucosa.

At our institution we prefer a combine technique that include nebulize local anesthetic with lidocaine 5% for 15–20 min beforehand and "spray as you-go" via the Fiberoptic bronchoscope working channel once the supraglottic structures are visible then wait another 1–3 min before intubation. This technique could be use via nasal or oral route.

Nerve block is the fastest way to achieve adequate airway anesthesia if time is a concern and it need smaller volume of local anesthetic. Using ultrasound guided technique could accelerate even more the process and success rate but it is a technique that need to be learned and master before trying it in the emergency room. Description of this technique it is beyond the objective of this chapter and can be available in several books and publications.

The mayor risk of local anesthetic is systemic toxicity, and it could lead to cardiovascular or neurologic impairment that also could be affected in these patients. Some

Drug	Dosing	Onset	Tachycardia	Antisialagogue	Sedation
Atropine	0.4–0.6 mg IV or IM 7 to 10 μg/kg IV	1 min (IV), 15–20 min (IM)	++++	++	+ Delirium (elderly)
Glycopyrrolate	0.2–0.3 mg IV or IM 7 to 10 μg/kg IV	1–2 min (IV), 20–30 min (IM)	+++	+++	—
Scopolamine	0.4 mg IV or IM	5–10 min (IV), 30–60 min (IM)	+	+++	+++

Abbreviation: IV, intravascular; IM, intramuscular; Min, minutes.

Table 2.
Summary of commonly used antimuscarinic drugs and they principal characteristics.

authors are limited the total dose to 9 mg • kg [8] but we recommend that dose should be kept between 3 and 5 mg • kg, especially in the critically ill but with stable conditions.

Gastric reflux is another mayor concern in these patients and can lead to bronchial aspiration and pneumonitis [19]. Medications like Histamine H2 blocker, Proton pump inhibitor and gastrointestinal tract (GI) pro-kinetics are commonly used. H2 receptor blocker routinely used are cimetidine 300 mg and ranitidine 50 mg and work by decreasing gastric acidity and volume, with a peak effect within 30–60 min [13, 19]. At our institution they have been stop used routinely because of side effect like gynecomastia (cimetidine) or risk of gastric cancer (ranitidine). Proton pump inhibitor such as omeprazole (40 mg iv) may have the same mechamism as H2 receptor blockers and has gain popularity and replace H2 receptor blocker at our institution, GI track pro-kinetics increase gastric emptying by increasing motility and can also increase lower esophageal sphincter tone, Metoclopramide 10 mg IV is the drug of choice, the risk of extrapyramidal syndrome has limited is use in Parkinson disease patients.

Sedation and hypnosis have become an essential part, same as local anesthetics in the preparation of awake tracheal intubation. Allowing a less traumatic experience for the patient by decreasing the level of stress also for the operator. Not all patients would tolerate some of the recommended medication, even with smaller doses, and could increase the incidence of undesirable side effects like bradycardia, hypoxia, dyspnea and cardiac or ventilatory failure. It's important to select the right patient and start at the minimal required dose of the medication titrated to adequate condition based on clinical signs [19]. These drugs are divided in several groups base on their clinical effects, anxiolysis (decrease anxiety), hypnosis (causes sleep or sedation) and analgesia (inhibit pain), they can be use alone or in combination. For anxiolysis the drugs of choice are Benzodiazepines and are the most popular used one in the emergency room, sometime there are the only medications used in preparation of awake tracheal intubation. Midazolam 0.5–1 mg IV or 0.07–0.1 mg · kg IM [19] have a rapid onset of time and shorter duration of action if administered intravascularly. Diazepam and Lorazepam are other drugs commonly but have a slower onset time and longer duration of action. Hypnosis could be accomplished by intravenous medication like Propofol and alpha 2 agonist like Dexmedetomidine. Propofol is a GABAergic central hypnotic, mostly popular among anesthesiologist but less used in other areas like the emergency department. Starting at a low bolus 30–50 mg and repeatedly over a period of 3–5 min until clinical effect, when combine with local anesthetic and analgesics and topicalization, could set the patient in good intubating condition with out overdosing. This will depend on clinical status and it's does not recommend if patient is unstable cardiopulmonary. Ketamine is another intravenous hypnotic and lately as gained popularity in emergency room awake intubation because of some advantages over Propofol. It causes hypnosis, but also increases blood pressure and heart rate by increasing blood catecholamines, it also has analgesics effects. Despite all these effects, caution should be taken when using this drug because of common side effect like increase intracranial pressure, increased salivation and bronchi reactivity leading to airway closure laryngospasm and bronchospasm [21]. Recommendations are to start with low dose boluses, 50 mg, titrated to clinical effects, also in combination of antisialagogues, more potent analgesics like opioids and bronchodilator like Salbutamol inhaled [2, 21]. We do not recommend infusion dose of Ketamine because of increased risk of mentioned side effects.

Alpha 2 agonist like Dexmedetomidine an imidazole compound as become the sedative/hypnotics of choice when performing an ATI outside the operating room in ambulatory seatings [8]. This because in a couple of minutes could cause adequate intubating conditions without compromising the respiratory system. It also has low analgesics effect, and in combination of other analgesics could potentiate this effect. Cautions should be taken because of reported severe bradycardia which has led to cardiac arrest. Recommended doses are an initial boluses 0.7–1 mcg · kg over a period of 10–15 min followed by a continuous infusion at a rate of 0.2–0.6 mcg · kg · h [8].

Opioids have been excellent adjuvant in controlling pain and anxiety during ATI, they principal mechanism is blocking opioid receptors in the central and peripheral nervous system [13]. Fentanyl and Remifentanyl are commonly used because of rapid onset and shorter duration of action. Remifentanyl it is metabolized by nonspecific plasma esterases, making it a good agent for continuous infusion during the procedure [19]. Recommended regimes vary, a dosing strategy could be as fallow a bolus of 0.5 μg/kg followed by an infusion of 0.1 μg/kg/min then gradually titrated by 0.025 to 0.05 μg/kg/min. The authors favor target control infusion using the Minto or Eleveld pharmacokinetics models, targeting a site effect concentration between of 0.15–0.25 ng/mL [19].

Combination of various drug is a common practice; at our institution we use a combination of Dexmedetomidine and ketamine. Finally, when selecting a drug always consider it's benefit base on patient individual clinical situation and hemodynamics.

4. Step by step approach

Clinical practice guidelines are a set of expert's recommendations and consensus often divided in related topics. They are not recipes and are subject to be accepted, modify, or rejected [22]. They must be adapted to local situation and available resources. Checklists are step-by-step approach that accelerate and facilitate repetitive processes, providing an outline for each participant.

The Difficult Airway Society guidelines for ATI are an excellent example [2], it provides an evidence-based summary of some of the relevant topics mentioned above in this chapter. It uses cognitive aid like visual aid infographic and pneumonic like the **sTOP technique**, which consist of several steps define by letters.

The first letter, the ′**s**′ mean sedation and can use any of the drugs mentioned earlier in the equipment and materials section of this chapter, it is written in lower case because it is an "optional" step and can be avoided or use at any time before the procedure.

The second letter ′ **T** ′ stand for Topicalization and it's the process of applying local anesthetics to numb the airway mucosa and allow procedure with mild discomfort for the patient. Most of the time we assess effectiveness based on patient report of heaviness or numbness of the oropharynx, but guideline recommend introducing object like suction or aspirations oral cannula to adequate good topicalization before procedure.

The third letter ′**O**′ it's an essential part and it's stand for oxygenation; comparison has demonstrated that of high flow nasal oxygen (> 30 L · min) have more effectiveness based on low desaturation incidents and expert recommendations. Use of supplemental oxygen is highly recommended by expert around the world and should be continue through the process of ATI.

The last letter '**P**' stand for the procedure of introducing the endotracheal tube and it finish once confirmation is assessed by two steps; visualize above the carina and capnography [8].

5. Complications

A traumatic procedure with or without bleeding, multiple attempts and failure to intubate can increase anxiety for the patient and the operator. Popular recommendation is to stop and analyze what step is the most difficult one and what changes should be made before attempting another try. If difficulty is the procedure itself, then it is better to handle it to a more experienced clinician.

Remember that the more attempt, this my cause mucosal edema that can lead to more obstruction. Attempt should be limited to three and advancing to another technique or equipment should be considered, like the use of supraglottic device, like laryngeal mask airway (LMA) and surgical airway front of neck airway (FONA), to maintain adequate ventilation and oxygenation.

6. Postprocedural care

Once confirmation that the endotracheal tube is in the right place and appropriately secure to the face; preparation for transferring to another area should be planned before. Patient should be anesthetized or deepen the sedation level and the administration of muscle relaxant should not delay; except they are contraindicated. Hemodynamic should be stable and monitoring like oxygen saturation (O2 sat), electrocardiogram (EKG), capnography and non-invasive blood pressure (NIBP).

7. Conclusions

Successful ATI should not be attempted alone, success is based on teamwork, good communication and patient cooperation.

A stepwise approach may reduce the incidence of failure and can assist the operator in finding difficult step.

Complication can occur and all emergency physicians should be prepared; calling for help in advance and maintain surgical doctor close by in case awake tracheostomy is need.

Author details

Erick Dunkley-Pinnock[1,2]

1 Pemex Regional Hospital, Reynosa, Tamaulipas, Mexico

2 Tamaulipas Autonomous University, Mexico

*Address all correspondence to: erick.dunkley@pemex.com

References

[1] Awake and Facilitated Intubations-USF Emergency Medicine. [Online]. Available: https://www.tampaemergencymedicine.org/blog/awake-and-facilitated-intubations-the-often-forgotten-option-in-our-airway-toolbox

[2] Ahmad I *et al.*. "Difficult Airway Society guidelines for awake tracheal intubation (ATI) in adults." Anaesthesia. Apr 2020;**75**(4):509–528. DOI: 10.1111/anae.14904

[3] James CDT. Sir William Macewen. Proceedings of the Royal Society of Medicine. 1974;**67**(4):237-242. DOI: 10.1177/003591577406700401

[4] Goksu S, Sen E. History of intubation. Journal of Academic Emergency Medicine. 2015;**14**(1):35-36. DOI: 10.5152/jaem.2015.96720

[5] Szmuk P, Ezri T, Evron S, Roth Y, Katz J. A brief history of tracheostomy and tracheal intubation, from the bronze age to the space age. Intensive Care Medicine. 2008;**34**(2):222-228. DOI: 10.1007/s00134-007-0931-5

[6] Collins SR, Blank RS. Fiberoptic intubation: An overview and update. American Association for Respiratory Care. 2014;**2014**:865-880. DOI: 10.4187/respcare.03012

[7] Apfelbaum JL et al. "2022 American Society of Anesthesiologists Practice Guidelines for Management of the Difficult Airway." Anesthesiology. Jan 2022;**136**(1):31–81. DOI: 10.1097/ALN.0000000000004002

[8] Leslie D, Stacey M. "Awake intubation," Continuing Education in Anaesthesia. Critical Care and Pain. Apr. 2015;**15**(2):64–67. DOI: 10.1093/bjaceaccp/mku015

[9] Kaisler MC, Hyde RJ, Sandefur BJ, Kaji AH, Campbell RL, Driver BE. Brown CA 3rd. Awake intubations in the emergency department: A report from the National Emergency Airway Registry. American Journal of Emergency Medicine. Nov 2021;**49**:48-51. DOI: 10.1016/j.ajem.2021.05.038. Epub 2021 May 15. PMID: 34062317

[10] Vissers RJ, Gibbs MA. The high-risk airway. Emergency Medicine Clinics of North America. 2010;**28**(1):203-217. DOI: 10.1016/j.emc.2009.10.004

[11] Law JA, Morris I, Kovacs G. Airway interventions and management in emergencies awake airway management and flexible endoscopic intubation key points. [Online]. Available: http://aimeairway.ca/book/

[12] Knudsen K, Nilsson U, Högman M, Pöder U. Awake intubation creates feelings of being in a vulnerable situation but cared for in safe hands: A qualitative study. BMC Anesthesiology. 2016;**16**(1). DOI: 10.1186/s12871-016-0240-z

[13] Ramkumar V. "Preparation of the patient and the airway for awake intubation." Indian Journal of Anaesthesia. Sep 2011;**55**(5):442–447. DOI: 10.4103/00195049.89863

[14] Dominguez N et al. Difficult airway in patients with head and neck masses a case description. AnesthesiologyNews.com. September 11, 2015. Available from: https://www.anesthesiologynews.com/Review-Articles/Article/08-15/Difficult-Airway-in-Patients-With-Head-or-Neck-Masses/33264

[15] Bradley P, Chapman G, Crooke B, Greenland K. ANZCA. 2016. Available from: https://aam.ucsf.edu/sites/g/files/tkssra4826/f/PU-Airway-Assessment-20160916v1.pdf

[16] Wong J, Lee JSE, Wong TGL, Iqbal R, Wong P. Fibreoptic intubation in airway management: A review article. Singapore Medical Journal. 2019;**60**(3):110-118. DOI: 10.11622/smedj.2018081

[17] Moore A, Schricker T. Awake videolaryngoscopy versus fiberoptic bronchoscopy. Current Opinion in Anaesthesiology. December 2019;**32**(6):764-768. DOI: 10.1097/ACO.0000000000000771

[18] Desai N, Ratnayake G, Onwochei DN, El-Boghdadly K, Ahmad I. Airway devices for awake tracheal intubation in adults: a systematic review and network meta-analysis. British Journal of Anaesthesia. 2021;**127**(4):636-647. DOI: 10.1016/j.bja.2021.05.025

[19] Artime CA, Sanchez A. Preparation of the patient for awake intubation | Clinical Gate. Available: https://clinicalgate.com/preparation-of-the-patient-for-awake-intubation/

[20] Han C et al. Improving mucosal anesthesia for awake endotracheal intubation with a novel method: A prospective, assessor-blinded, randomized controlled trial. BMC Anesthesiology. 2020;**20**(1). DOI: 10.1186/s12871-020-01210-8

[21] Parks A, O'connell K, Hoang R. Wake Up! Awake Intubation in the ED. 2019. [Online]. Available: https://emottawablog.com/2019/10/wake-up-awake-intubation-in-the-ed/1/8

[22] Franco JVA, Arancibia M, Meza N, Madrid E, Kopitowski K. Guías de práctica clínica: conceptos, limitaciones y desafíos. Medwave. 2020;**20**(3):e7887. DOI: 10.5867/medwave.2020.03.7887

Chapter 6

Extubations Protocols in the Neurocritical Patient

Jorge Francisco Piña Rubio, María Elena Buenrostro Espinosa, Ricardo Serrano Tamayo, Jesus Cuevas Garcia, Ana Valentina Plascencia Gutiérrez, José David Durán Morales and Larry Chavira Calderon

Abstract

Within neurosurgical procedures, it has been observed that the failure rate covers up to 70%. It has been observed that early extubation has been associated with a decrease in mortality as well as a shorter hospital stay. Delaying extubation to obtain sustained neurological improvement during the recovery phase does not guarantee successful extubation. Studies have observed that up to 80% of patients with Glasgow less than 8 have been successfully extubated. It must be remembered that the Glasgow scale does not assess the difference in disorders of consciousness nor does it evaluate stem reflexes in intubated patients, so current studies have opted for other scales that allow us to assess the state of consciousness with more criteria to evaluate. It is demonstrated that the delay in extubation for neurological recovery did not show successful extubation and was associated with an increase in nosocomial pneumonia, longer stay in the ICU, and hospital cost. It is important to emphasize the evaluation of this type of patients, placing special emphasis on the cardiac and pulmonary repercussions of patients who suffer neurological lesions, since alterations that could go unnoticed could mean a failure to extubation with repercussions on the morbidity and mortality of patients.

Keywords: extubation, neurocritical patient, neurological assessment, extubation protocols, delay extubation

1. Introduction

In neurosurgical procedures, it has been observed that the rate of extubation failure covers up to 70%. It is important to seek early extubation, since it has currently been associated with a decrease in mortality and a shorter hospital stay.

Within the extubation criteria we have that adequate hemodynamic and ventilatory status are important for the patient. The approach to ventilatory aspects emphasizes adequate oxygenation and lung function, while in hemodynamic aspects, patients must always have an adequate balance of this, without the support of any vasopressor.

One of the main objectives of this chapter is the approach to the neurocritical patient. For some time it has been observed that the majority of patients admitted for neurosurgical procedures are maintained under orotracheal intubation by mechanical ventilation regardless of the neurological etiology, the surgical procedure and the anesthetic management.

Today, the use of neuromonitoring is essential in all patients undergoing neurological surgery, and this guides us on the maintenance of intracranial pressure, cerebral perfusion and cerebral oxygen consumption, in order to carry out adequate extubation in neurocritical patients.

At the same time, an adequate pre-anesthetic evaluation is of vital importance to know the patient undergoing surgery, where the type of procedure is evaluated, the approach and to know if there is any cardiac or pulmonary repercussion that could lead to a failed extubation and thus be able to maintain our neurosurgical patient extubation protocol in the best conditions.

2. Epidemiology

The main causes leading to advanced airway management in neurological patients are cerebrovascular event (CVD), whether of ischemic or hemorrhagic origin, head trauma (TBI), subarachnoid hemorrhage, and parenchymal hemorrhage. It has been proven that prolonged mechanical ventilation after orotracheal intubation is associated with pneumonia, venous thrombosis, increased hospital stay, and worse clinical prognosis [1]. Friedman [2] carried out a study where he analyzed the complications of patients with subarachnoid hemorrhage secondary to an aneurysm and concluded that patients with pulmonary complications had a worse prognosis than those who did not have this alteration. He, in turn, also found that patients with prolonged intubation had more complications at the pulmonary level [2]. TCE has remained a serious health problem worldwide. Annually it is estimated that there are 10 million TCEs that lead to death or hospitalization. In the United States, the average ranges from 1.4 million per year, reaching a mortality of up to 50,000 patients [3].

Currently, neurosurgical teams and neuroanesthesiologists have focused on the search for safe extubation protocols for neurocritical patients and avoid the previously mentioned complications in these patients.

3. Content

Within the area of neurocritical patients we have different terms that should be mentioned.

- Delayed extubation is defined as those patients who have not been extubated in the first 48 hours; a rate of 30% is currently estimated in neurocritical patients.

- Failed extubation is seen when there is a need to reintubate and resume treatment with ventilatory support between 24 and 72 hours after the removal of the tracheal tube.

- Early extubation is mentioned as the transition from mechanical ventilation of a patient to spontaneous ventilation within the first 6–8 hours after surgery.
- The term Ultra fast track is when the patient is extubated in the operating room, terms that have been described in cardiology surgery [4].

It is worth mentioning that the term Ultra fast track is mainly attributed to early extubation in patients undergoing cardiac surgery, and has gained importance since the 1950s, since due to the lack of adequate equipment and personnel in care units Intensive care, the lack of mechanical ventilation providers, and the long stays of patients with unfavorable prognoses, patients were subjected to early extubation to avoid complications resulting from poor postoperative management. However, these presented serious complications such as severe hypoxemia, acidosis, which led to death, derived from poor management in extubation, so that in the mid-70s, patients in the postoperative period remained under Mechanic Ventilation with better criteria. and handling that paradoxically favored its prognosis. The rapid evolution of cardiovascular sciences led to an increase in the number of patient care, so new programs were implemented that benefited the study of the Fast Track extubation technique, to reduce hospital stays and today it is one of the techniques of extubation with a greater number of study protocols and validation in the postoperative management of patients with heart disease [5].

However, in the area of neuroanesthesia, there is a huge lack of studies and protocols that benefit or indicate the safest tools to take, when faced with whether or not to extubate a patient.

At the moment of having any alteration at the level of the central nervous system, the awake state is reduced and induces patients to present hypoventilation, which can lead to bronchial aspiration. One of the first measures has been to support the airway with orotracheal intubation. Goals for adequate cerebral blood flow should be maintained in all neurological patients. These include treatment of hypoxemia with PaO_2 targets greater than 60 mmHg, control of $PaCO_2$ of 32–45 mmHg, as well as adequate cerebral perfusion pressure between 50 and 150 mmHg. Due to the great complications that are obtained in patients with extubation failure, the fear of extubation has been the subject of controversy regarding when to withdraw ventilatory support.

The Glasgow coma scale in the neurocritical patient has been used as a criterion for extubation; currently, delaying extubation to obtain neurological improvement during the recovery phase does not guarantee successful extubation. Studies have observed that up to 80% of patients with Glasgow less than 8 have been successfully extubated. It must be remembered that this scale does not assess stalk reflexes in intubated patients. At present, other scales have been evaluated that allow us to assess the awake state in the neurosurgical patient with more precision.

Karim Asehnoune evaluated the predictors of extubation in patients with brain damage in a multicenter study. A total of 437 patients were included using the VISAGE score (visual pursuit, swallowing, age, Glasgow for extubation) (**Table 1**).

This score was used to assess the success rate in extubation where those patients with a score of 0 had a 23% extubation rate, a score of 1 with 56% extubation, and it was significantly higher in patients with a score of 2–3 (70–90% extubation).

Extubation success score	Assigned points according to items
Age < 40 yr old (yes/no)	1/0
Visual pursuit (yes/no)	1/0
Swallowing attempts (yes/no)	1/0
Glasgow coma score > 10 (yes/no)	1/0
VISAGE = visual pursuit, swallowing, age, Glasgow for extubation	

This is an author's work Asehnoune et al. [6].

Table 1.
VISAGE score.

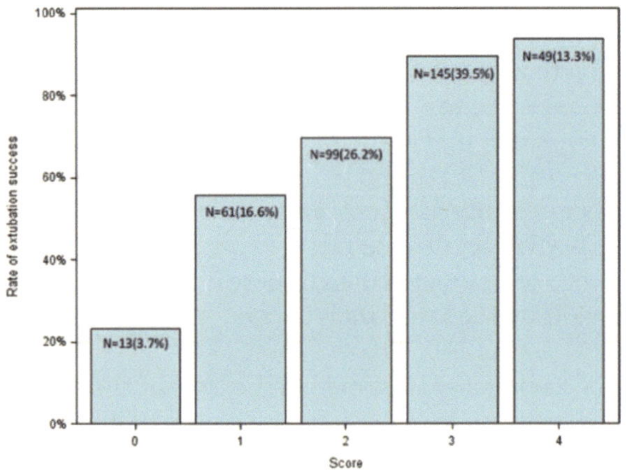

Figure 1.
Rate of extubation success according to the number of predictive factors. This is an author's work Asehnoune et al. [6].

Score equal to or greater than 3 predict extubation success with a sensitivity of 62% and a specificity of 79% (**Figure 1**).

In this study, the main cause of brain damage was traumatic brain injury and this, in turn, had the highest rate of extubation. The main causes of extubation failure were neurological disorders, hypoxemia, mismanagement of endotracheal secretions, cardiovascular failure, and postextubation stridor [5].

In 2021, the PRICE (Predicting Intratentorial Craniotomy Extubation) survey was conducted with 5453 physicians responsible for neurosurgical management. These surveys were addressed to Neuroanesthesiologists, Neurointensivists and Neurosurgeons whose primary objective was to estimate extubation times in neurosurgical patients and assess their prognosis. It was found that the proportion of patients with extubation at the end of the surgical procedure was higher in high-volume centers compared to low-volume centers and that the anesthesiology service was the service that had the highest extubation of neurosurgical patients together with support. of neurosurgeons. The main factors associated with not performing an early extubation were based on the course of the surgical procedure, the patient's awake state and if he presented any alteration at the bulbar level (**Figure 2**).

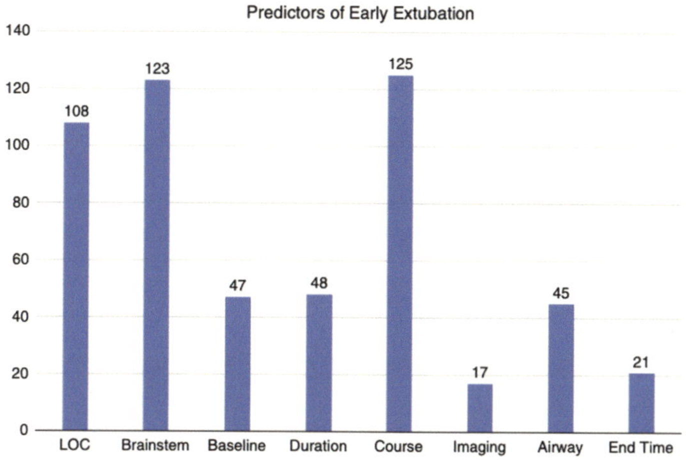

Figure 2.
Predictors selected by respondents to identify candidates for early extubation after elective infratentorial craniotomy. Airway indicates suspicion or history of difficult airway management; baseline, patient's physical status before surgery; brainstem, evidence of bulbar dysfunction; course, course of surgery; duration, duration of surgery; end time, the time of day when surgery ends; imaging, preoperative imaging; LOC, level of consciousness. This is an author's work Gaudet et al. [7].

It was concluded that the decision for early extubation should be made maintaining adequate communication between neurosurgeons, neuroanesthesiologists and neurointensivists, as well as adequate clinical knowledge of the patient prior to the surgical event [4].

Within the extubation criteria are goals based on hemodynamic, ventilatory and neurological patterns.

One of the neurological parameters that has been used is the Glasgow coma scale, Coplin et al., demonstrated that the delay in extubation for neurological recovery did not show successful extubation and was associated with an increase in nosocomial pneumonia, longer stay in the ICU and hospital cost [7]. We know that the Glasgow coma scale assesses the motor, speech and visual area, but one of its main limitations is that it cannot be assessed in a patient under ventilatory support, since it does not differentiate between the patient's waking state disorders, does not it assesses stem reflexes and is primarily not useful in the patient under orotracheal intubation [8].

A possible alternative is to use the Coma Recovery Scale-Revised, which offers us a more extensive evaluation, assessing auditory function, visual function, motor function, oromotor or verbal function, communication capacity, and ability to wake up. Chatelle et al. describe the scale as being more comprehensive and capable of better detecting a patient's awake state (**Figure 3**) [9].

Bodien et al., carried out a statistical analysis about the sensitivity and specificity of the Coma Recovery Scale-Revised to adequately detect and identify the state of consciousness of the patient and through a ROC (Receiver Operating Characteristic) analysis, they found an area under the curve of 0.98, which far exceeds the 0.681 of the Glasgow Coma Scale, which was reported by Namen et al. [9, 10] (**Figure 4**).

In order to establish an adequate extubation protocol in neurosurgical patients, spontaneous breathing test maneuvers must be taken into account, such as the T-piece test, continuous positive airway pressure (CPAP) with levels equal to those of pressure positive end-expiratory and invasive ventilation with low level pressure support (5–8 cmH_2O) or automatic tube compensation [11].

Table 1 Coma Recovery Scale-Revised

Score	Test
Auditory function scale	
4	Consistent movement to command*
3	Reproducible movement to command*
2	Localization to sound
1	Auditory startle
0	None
Visual function scale	
5	Object recognition*
4	Object localization: reaching*
3	Visual pursuit*
2	Fixation*
1	Visual startle
0	None
Motor function scale	
6	Functional object use†
5	Automatic motor response*
4	Object manipulation*
3	Localization to noxious stimulation*
2	Flexion withdrawal
1	Abnormal posturing
0	None/flaccid
Oromotor/verbal function scale	
3	Intelligible verbalization*
2	Vocalization/oral movement
1	Oral reflexive movement
0	None
Communication scale	
2	Functional: accurate†
1	Nonfunctional: intentional*
0	None
Arousal scale	
3	Attention
2	Eye opening without stimulation
1	Eye opening with stimulation
0	Unarousable

* Indicates a minimally conscious state.
† Indicates emergence from the minimally conscious state.

Figure 3.
Parameters evaluated by the Coma Recovery Scale-Revised that make it possible to identify the state of consciousness of a patient. This is an author's work Chatelle et al. [9].

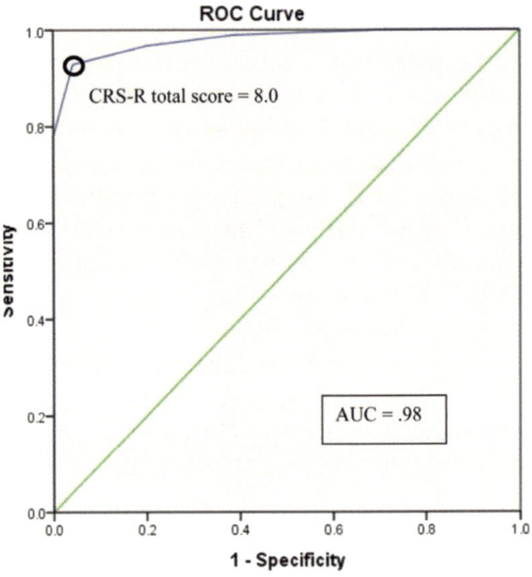

Figure 4.
ROC analysis to identify the sensitivity of the Coma Recovery Scale-Revised to adequately identify the states of consciousness of patients. This is an author's work Bodien et al. [10].

Navalesi and Frigerio analyzed the reintubation rate in neurological patients in the intensive care unit based on the following criteria: Glasgow coma scale greater than 8, presence of audible cough during suction, normal serum Na, core temperature less than 38.5°C, pH greater than 7.35, $PaCO_2$ less than 50 mm Hg or PAO_2/FiO_2 greater than 200 with positive end-expiratory pressure less than 5 cm H_2O, FiO_2 less than 0.4, heart rate less than 125 beats per minute, and systolic blood pressure greater at 90 mmHg without norepinephrine or epinephrine support. These patients were compared against a control group managed by different physicians with personal criteria for weaning from mechanical ventilation.

Both groups were analyzed and it was observed that the reintubation rate was 12% in the control group while 5% was manifested in the intervention group with the aforementioned criteria, concluding that those patients with neurological disorders who are taken with adequate both clinical and physiological objectives can improve outcomes and decrease the rate of reintubation in intensive care patients [12].

Bösel [14] published an algorithm about which patients are safe to perform extubation (in patients with neurological pathology in intensive care), if we analyze the criteria made by Navalesi and Frigerio we can see that the hemodynamic, ventilatory and neurological variables are very similar, with the exception that Bosel considers that time is a fundamental variable for performing an early tracheostomy and thus avoiding the risk of reintubation (**Figure 5**) [13].

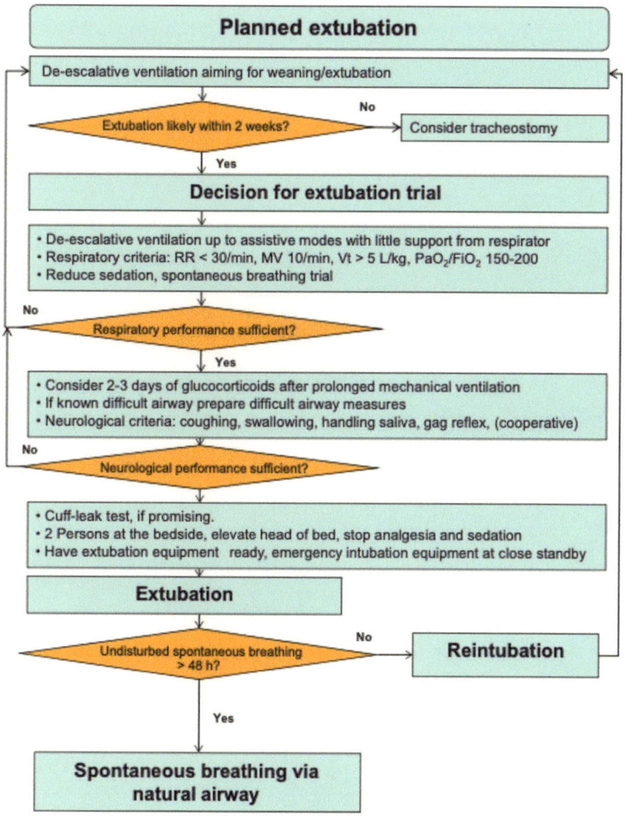

Figure 5.
Suggestion for approaching extubation in the neuroscience intensive care unit. This is an author's work Bösel [14].

Grade	Cough during the aspiration maneuver	Number of secretions (need for passes)	Color of secretions	Viscosity of secretions	Interval of aspiration of secretions	Vomiting reflex
0	Vigorous	0	Clear	Aqueous	More than 3 h	Vigorous
1	Moderate	1	Clear brown	Frothy	Every 2–3 h	Moderate
2	Weak	2	Yellow	Dense	Every 1–2 h	Weak
3	Absent	≥3	Green	Sticky	<1 h	Absent

This is an author's work Jibaja et al. [15].

Table 2.
Airway care score.

Another piece of information included in the M. Jibaja algorithm is the Airway care score, which is useful for predicting the ability to maintain a safe airway (**Table 2**).

With this score, once the patients met the prerequisites to be able to be extubated, they analyzed the values and if they were above 7, the algorithm tells us to look for some etiology as a trigger for the ventilatory cause. If it was less than 7, the already established extubation criteria were used (**Figure 6**) [14].

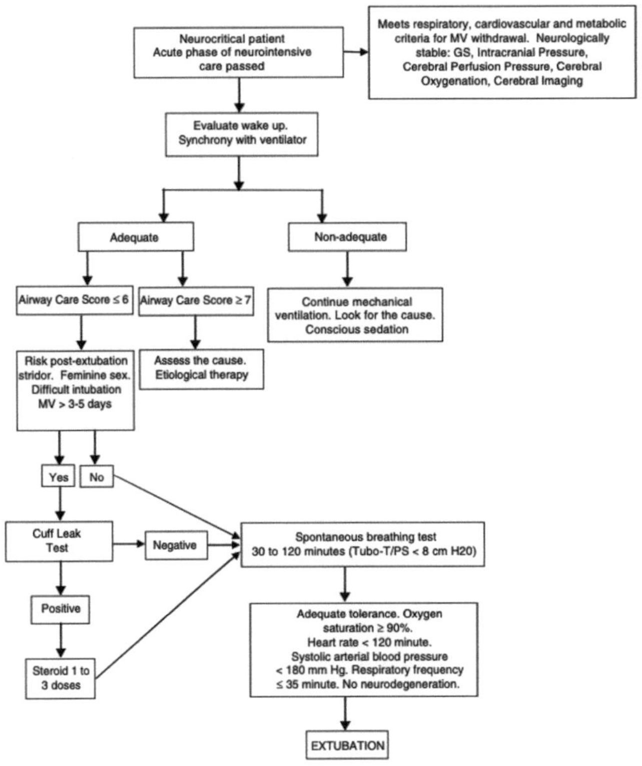

Figure 6.
Algorithm for weaning from MV and extubation in neurocritical patients. This is an author's work Jibaja et al. [15].

Extubation criteria in posterior fossa surgery		
Ventilation-oxygenation	**Hemodynamics**	**Neurological**
Respiratory rate 10–30 breaths per minute	Cardiovascular stability	GCS > 8 points
Regular respiratory pattern	Lack of dependency of vasoactive agents	Adequate psychological conditions
Max inspiratory pressure < 20 cmH_2O	Temperature 35–37°C	Lack of depression of the respiratory center due anesthetics
Tidal volume > 6 ml/kg	Heart rate < 100 bpm	Integrity of the protective airway reflexes
FIO_2 < 50%	MAP > 65 mmHg	Nausea reflex (IX, X)
Intrapulmonar shunt (Qs/Qt < 20%)	PH 7.35–7.45	Faringeal reflex (cough) (V, X)
PaO_2 > 70 mmHg	HB >8 g/dL	Vocal folds mobility (X)
$PaCO_2$ 30–45 mmHg	Urine output >1 ml/kg/h	Integrity of the greater hypoglossal nerve (tongue movements, strength by palpation)
PaO_2/FIO_2 > 200	ICP < 15 mmHg	Reversal of the neuromuscular block

This is an author's work De La Serna-Soto et al. [4].

Table 3.
Extubation criteria in posterior fossa surgery.

Another aspect that must be taken into account is the type of neurosurgical procedure to be performed. We know that infratentorial injuries, as discussed in the PRICE survey, are a challenge for neurosurgeons, neuroanesthesiologists, and neurointensivists, and this is due to the fact that infratentorial injuries have a higher rate of failed extubation, prolonged mechanical ventilation, pneumonia, high mortality, and increased hospital costs. Cai, assessed that lesions greater than 30 mm, which are associated with low torque dysfunction, patients with a history of previous craniotomy and sudden changes in blood pressure, were the main predictors of extubation failure in neurosurgical patients [6, 15, 16].

At the National Institute of Neurology and Neurosurgery of Mexico, criteria for extubation in patients undergoing posterior fossa surgery were analyzed and described in **Table 3** [4].

4. Conclusions

It must be taken into account that there are complications associated with the delay and failure of extubation in neurocritical patients, which is why all patients must be evaluated in detail prior to surgical intervention. The neurological examination is essential to know the state prior to the surgical procedure. We know that there are different extubation protocols for neurocritical patients and all of them should be reviewed in detail for a better prognosis. In turn, infratentorial lesions have a higher risk of extubation failure and that is why we must analyze and detail an adequate clinical history in our patient. Since there is not enough evidence for the extubation of these patients, the global implementation of extubation guidelines for neurocritical patients is recommended.

Author details

Jorge Francisco Piña Rubio[1,2]*, María Elena Buenrostro Espinosa[3,4], Ricardo Serrano Tamayo[5,6], Jesus Cuevas Garcia[6,7], Ana Valentina Plascencia Gutiérrez[8,9], José David Durán Morales[2,8] and Larry Chavira Calderon[2,8]

1 Neurological Anesthesia, Mexicali, Baja California, Mexico

2 Hospital General de Mexicali, Mexico

3 Oncological Anesthesia, Mexicali, Baja California, Mexico

4 IMSS Hospital Regional de Especialidades No. 30, Mexico

5 Neurological Anesthesia, Mexico City, Mexico

6 Hospital General Ajusco Medio, Neurological Anesthesia, CDMX, Mexico

7 Centro Médico Nacional 20 Noviembre ISSSTE, Mexico

8 Anesthesia Resident, Mexicali, Baja California, Mexico

9 ISSSTE Hospital General 5 de Diciembre, Mexico

*Address all correspondence to: jfrancisco.pina@hotmail.com

References

[1] Tanwar G, Singh U, Kundra S, Chaudhary AK, Sunil Kaytal AG. Evaluation of airway care score as a criterion for extubation in patients admitted in neurosurgery intensive care unit. Journal of Anaesthesiology Clinical Pharmacology. 2018;**34**(3):46-50

[2] Friedman JA, Pichelmann MA, Piepgras DG, McIver JI, Toussaint LG, McClelland RL, et al. Pulmonary complications of aneurysmal subarachnoid hemorrhage. Neurosurgery. 2003;**52**(5):1025-1032

[3] Langlois JA, Rutland-Brown W, Wald MM. The epidemiology and impact of traumatic brain injury: A brief overview. The Journal of Head Trauma Rehabilitation. 2006;**21**(5):375-378

[4] De J, Serna-Soto L, Osorio-Santiago A, Manrique-Carmona P. Articulo de revisión Cirugía de fosa posterior y extubación fallida. Anestesia en México. 2, mayo-agosto. 2017;**29**:1-6

[5] Bruder N, Ravussin P. Recovery from anesthesia and postoperative extubation of neurosurgical patients: A review. Journal of Neurosurgical Anesthesiology. 1999;**11**:282-293

[6] Asehnoune K, Seguin P, Lasocki S, Roquilly A, Delater A, Gros A, et al. Extubation success prediction in a multicentric cohort of patients with severe brain injury. Anesthesiology. 2017;**127**(2):338-346

[7] Gaudet JG, Levy CS, Jakus L, Goettel N, Meling TR, Quintard H. Early extubation after elective infratentorial craniotomy: Results of the international PRICE survey. Journal of Neurosurgical Anesthesiology. 2022:1-5

[8] Coplin WM, Pierson DJ, Cooley KD, Newell DW, Rubenfeld GD. Implications of extubation delay in brain-injured patients meeting standard weaning criteria. American Journal of Respiratory and Critical Care Medicine. 2000;**161**(5):1530-1536

[9] Chatelle C, Bodien YG, Carlowicz C, Wannez S, Charland-Verville V, Gosseries O, et al. Detection and interpretation of impossible and improbable coma recovery scale-revised scores. Archives of Physical Medicine and Rehabilitation. 2016;**97**(8):1295-1300.e4. DOI: 10.1016/j.apmr.2016.02.009. Epub 2016 Mar 2. Erratum in: Arch Phys Med Rehabil. 2018 Dec;**99**(12):2649-2650

[10] Bodien YG, Carlowicz CA, Chatelle C, Giacino JT. Sensitivity and specificity of the Coma Recovery Scale–Revised Total Score in detection of conscious awareness. Archives of Physical Medicine and Rehabilitation. 2016;**97**(3):490-492.e1. DOI: 10.1016/j.apmr.2015.08.422. Epub 2015 Sep 3

[11] Namen AM, Ely EW, Tatter SB, Case LD, Lucia MA, Smith A, et al. Predictors of successful extubation in neurosurgical patients. American Journal of Respiratory and Critical Care Medicine. 2001;**163**(3 Pt 1):658-664. DOI: 10.1164/ajrccm.163.3.2003060

[12] Zein H, Baratloo A, Negida A, Safari S. Ventilator weaning and spontaneousbreathing trials; an educational review. Emergency. 2016;**4**(2):65-71

[13] Navalesi P, Frigerio P, Moretti MP, Sommariva M, Vesconi S, Baiardi P, et al. Rate of reintubation in mechanically ventilated neurosurgical and

neurologic patients: Evaluation of a systematic approach to weaning and extubation. Critical Care Medicine. 2008;**36**(11):2986-2992

[14] Bösel J. Who is safe to extubate in the neuroscience intensive care unit, Seminars in Respiratory and Critical Care Medicine. 2017;**38**(6):830-839

[15] Jibaja M, Sufan JL, Godoy DA. Controversies in weaning from mechanical ventilation and extubation in the neurocritical patient. Medicina Intensiva. 2018:**42**:551-555

[16] Cai YH, Wang HT, Zhou JX. Perioperative predictors of extubation failure and the effect on clinical outcome after infratentorial craniotomy. Medical Science Monitor. 2016;**22**:2431-2438

Chapter 7

Peri-Operative Management of a Difficult Airway in a Resource Limited Environment

Omolola Fagbohun

Abstract

Airway management is an essential skill that is relevant to the practice of medicine especially with regards specialties such as anesthesia, intensive care and emergency medicine. This vital skill can be made more challenging in an austere environment with limited facilities and equipment. Being pre-informed on the peculiarity of each patient, developing and mastering necessary skills through regular trainings and having a pre- outlined care plan based on available resources in the immediate environment can mitigate against some of the possible challenges in such environment. Hence, the pre-operative assessment of a patient with a difficult airway is an integral part of the peri-operative workup that helps to predict potential problems, develop a management plan thereby avoiding an unanticipated difficult airway as much as possible and inadvertently preparing for an unanticipated difficult airway in rare instances.

Keywords: difficult airway, limited resources, anticipated difficult airway, airway equipment, supraglottic devices, advanced airway equipment

1. Introduction

Airway management hazards are common causes of morbidity and mortality in the peri-operative period especially in a resource limited environment. Adequate airway assessment is essential in the care of all patients requiring advanced airway management. The goal of airway assessment is to identify patients who may have difficult airway and develop practical management options depending on the cause of the difficult airway, the patient's condition, skill of the attending airway manager and the available equipment in the immediate environment. There are two major focus areas in the management of a difficult airway:

a. Laryngoscopy and intubation

b. Ventilation (oxygenation)

Although protocols are available to guide the management of difficult airways, but these protocols can only help each team or unit to develop guidelines that are convenient and peculiar to them based on available equipment, skill of attending airway managers and the cause of difficulty in airway. The aim is to prevent critical airway outcomes such as hypoxic brain injury, cardiac arrest, oropharyngeal trauma and death. Predicting problems with ventilation and oxygenation supersedes predicting difficulties with laryngoscopy or intubation as failed laryngoscopy is not as dangerous as a situation of failed oxygenation. Airway assessment to predict a difficult airway will entail history taking, examination and investigations. For patients who have never been intubated, airway difficulty can only be suspected from review [1].

According to the American Society of Anaesthesiologists Task Force definitions [1]:

The difficult airway occurs when a conventionally trained Anesthetist has difficulty with either facemask or laryngeal mask airway ventilation, tracheal intubation or all the three clinical scenarios.

Problem with facemask ventilation is when the conventional anesthetist cannot maintain oxygen saturation on at least 92% as measured by a pulse oximeter or prevent clinical evidence of deficient ventilation during advanced airway management. With difficult laryngoscopy, a conventional anesthetist has a problem visualizing the vocal cords. This usually corresponds to a Cormack and Lehane Grade IV laryngoscopy view [1, 2].

A difficult intubation occurs when a conventional laryngoscopy requires more than three attempts or more than 10 minutes to introduce an endotracheal tube by a conventionally trained anesthetist.

The prevalence of difficult airways varies widely and changes with the environment, situation and type of patient. It is approximately1 in 1–2000 in the elective setting, 1 in 300 during rapid sequence intubation in the obstetric setting and 1 in 50–100 in the emergency department, intensive care unit, and pre-hospital settings [1, 3].

2. Identifying a Difficult Airway

The management of a difficult airway begins with the anticipation of a difficult airway and developing a plan to avert critical incidents due to a difficult airway encounter. The prediction of a difficult airway is heralded by a proper pre- operative assessment [1].

2.1 Pre-operative airway evaluation

This involves history taking, examination, investigation, familiarization with the work environment and available instruments to maneuver the airway, identifying the strength of each team member and assigning roles, identifying shortfalls and developing care plans that fits the immediate environment while not deviating from acceptable world standards [1, 3].

2.2 History

History that may suggest difficult airway management includes: The Reason for airway management, obesity, history suggestive of obstructive sleep apnea, exercise intolerance, smoking, change in voice, difficulty swallowing, burns affecting the airway, poor mouth opening, poor neck mobility, large mammary glands, Infections of the oropharynx and neck, previous surgery or radiotherapy to neck, difficult dentition, pregnancy, recent intubation (swelling, trauma), previous anesthetics and operations, previous difficulties with mask ventilation or laryngoscopy [4, 5].

2.3 Examination

The level of consciousness and co-operation, Body Mass Index, Beard, craniofacial deformity, Mallampati grade I to IV, Mouth opening, Inter-incisor gap distance (> 3 cm = good, < 3 cm = bad), Shape of palate, Jaw protrusion, Teeth, Edentuous, Teeth prominence (upper incisors) and condition, Relation of maxillary to mandibular incisors during normal jaw closure, dentures/ caps/ crowns/ loose teeth, Range of motion of head and neck, thyro-mental distance <6 cm, Neck length and circumference/ thickness, Compliance of mandibular space, Sternomental distance, upper lip bite test, Mallampati Classification [4, 5].

2.4 Investigations

- Nasal endoscopy, awake laryngoscopy, Lateral neck xray, Chest Xray, CT neck

2.5 Modified Mallampati score

- Class I: the soft palate, the uvula, fauces and pillars are seen easily [4]
- Class II: the soft palate, the uvula and the fauces are seen
- Class III: only the Soft palate and the base of the uvula can be seen
- Class IV: Only the hard palate can be seen

Class III/IV predicts a difficult airway. The mallampattit scoring system can not be used alone to predict difficulty [6, 7].

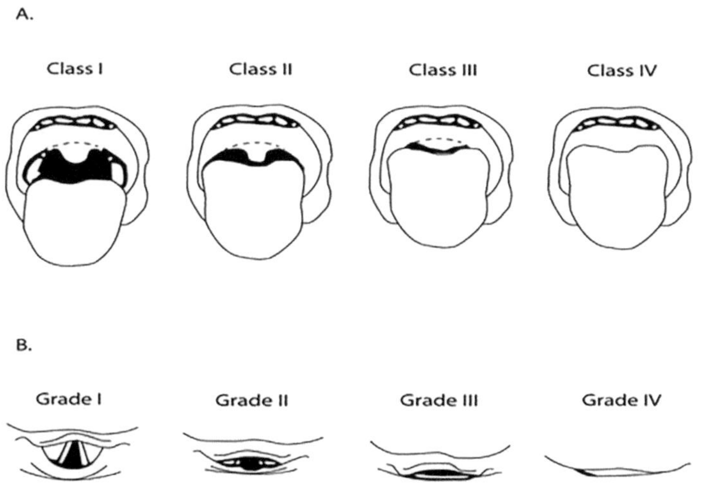

2.6 Cormack-Lehane classification

- Grade 1: The full glottis is seen
- Grade 2a: The glottis is partially seen
- Grade 2b: Only the posterior aspect of the glottis is seen
- Grade 3: Only epiglottis seen, no part of the glottis is sighted
- Grade 4: No part of the glottis or the epiglottis is seen

A difficult intubation is suggested with a Grade 2b view or more [2].

Upper Lip Bite Test [8]. The upper lip bite test assesses the ability to place the lower incisors over the mucosa of the upper lip. This acts as a predictor of the ability to subluxate the mandible during laryngoscopy. The grading system is as follows:

- Grade 1: the upper lip can be fully covered by the lower incisors
- Grade 2: the upper lip can be partially covered with the lower incisors
- Grade 3: the lower teeth cannot reach the upper lip [8]

3. Acronyms for difficult airway predictions

3.1 The acronym for difficult laryngoscopy and intubation is the LEMON SCORE

- Look externally for facial anomaly, bleeding, small mouth [9]
- Evaluate 3-3-2 rule
- Mallampati score
- Obstruction/ Obesity
- Neck Mobility for trauma, arthritis, spondylosis and consider the use of video laryngoscopy

3.2 The acronym for the Difficult Bag Valve Mask (BVM) ventilation is BONES

The difficult BVM is described according to the American Society of Anesthesiologists (ASA) as a situation in which it is impossible to provide adequate ventilation due to poor mask seal, excessive gas leak or excess resistance to gas inflow or outflow [9].

- Beard
- Obese

- No teeth
- Elderly
- Sleep Apnea / Snoring

3.3 The mnemonic for difficulty using a supra glottic device such as the laryngeal mask airway, LMA = RODS

- Restricted mouth opening [9]
- Obstruction
- Distorted or disrupted airway
- Stiff lungs or cervical-spine

3.4 The acronym for Difficult surgical airway (difficult cricothyrotomy) is SHORT

- Surgery or other airway obstruction [9]
- Hematoma, Infection or abcess
- Obesity
- Radiation distortion or other deformity
- Tumor

4. Strategy for managing a predicted difficult airway: A pre planned pre-induction strategy includes:

4.1 Familiarization with the procedural environment

Is the anesthetic team conversant with the procedural environment? Is it the regular theater. Emergency room, the intensive care unit or a totally strange environment like an accident point, a catheterization laboratory? Do they have all needed equipment and resuscitatory drugs available? Do they have adequate support staff? Do they need to move needed equipment such as back up laryngoscopes, difficult airway trolleys and others to augment the facilities where the procedure will take place [1].

4.2 Selection of equipment

The choice of appropriate airway device is essential for effective airway management. The use of the facemask, oropharyngeal airway, curved and straight-blade laryngoscopes, different sizes of endotracheal tubes with adequate airway training skills were the mainstay of endotracheal intubation and airway management. The facemask is a basic airway device for providing ventilation during airway management. This then led to the introduction of the gum-elastic bougie for accessing minimally visible laryngeal inlets even after applying significant externally applied downward and upward laryngeal pressure. The bougie is then serving as a guide for advancing the endotracheal tube. Endotracheal tubes are devices inserted through the nose or mouth to provide oxygenation and ventilation. The distal end of the tube is located at the mid-trachea [1, 8, 10].

When the facemask fails to provide adequate ventilation/oxygenation in some situations (such as craniofacial deformities, edentulousness) which may require filling the defect with gauzes to support holding the facemask or handling the facemask with special techniques and the larynx cannot be accessed with the external maneuver or a gum elastic bougie, the use of supra glottic airway adjuncts may be necessary. Supraglottic airways devices ventilate from above the glottis. A common supraglottic device used in airway management is the Laryngeal Mask Airway, LMA. LMAs are used during difficult facemask ventilation and they can be used during difficult intubation as conduits for introducing the endotracheal tube [8, 11].

The LMAs can be used for noninvasive positive-pressure ventilation to provide positive-pressure airway support. Patients can be placed on a continuous positive airway pressure (CPAP) device or a bilevel positive airway pressure (BIPAP) device. The noninvasive positive-pressure ventilation is ideal in conscious patients with ventilatory efforts. However, patient should be closely monitored for a decline in consciousness or depreciating respiratory effort or exhaustion so that endotracheal intubation is established if needed [12].

A supraglottic device may be considered in difficult mask ventilation or difficult intubation .cases, or when a rescue device or conduit is required for endotracheal tube introduction during difficult intubation. For a difficult intubation, the use of a gum elastic bougie, the intubating LMA, a video laryngoscope or awake fibreoptic intubation are the various options.

When a difficult airway is encountered, the downward and upward laryngeal pressure maneuver is performed to attempt to bring the laryngeal inlet into better view. The gum elastic bougie is used for accessing minimally visible laryngeal inlets after the above maneuver fails. The bougie serves as a guide to advance the endotracheal tube.

It is important to note that, the patient, the cause of difficulty, the skill of the anesthetist and the available equipment are all determinants of the choice of equipment and technique of airway management. The Intubating Laryngeal Mask Airway, ILMA is a special type of LMA that is recommended in the management of a difficult airway. It is said to have about 94% success rate [11].

The awake fibreoptic intubation is another option for managing a difficult airway. These are not readily available in resource limited facilities. Although studies have recorded 88–100% success rate in their use for managing difficult airways. The ILMA and the awake fibreoptic intubation are said to have comparable success rate [12].

The video laryngoscope is a choice equipment for managing a difficult airway. It enables smooth and safe introduction of eitheran endotracheal tube, an endotracheal tube introducer, or fiber optic scopes in the care of both an anatomically normal upper airways and also those with a difficult upper airway. The video laryngoscope has an in built camera that allows the process of airway management to be watched on a screen that is either attached to the handle of the laryngoscope itself or is freestanding. There are various types of video laryngoscopes offering different designs of laryngoscope blades such as the straight, curved or hyper-angulated blades [13, 14]. It is advisable that the managing anesthetist uses the equipment they are familiar with and they have available on their airway trolley arranged with available resuscitatory drugs. With a failed attempt at intubation despite the use of the LMA, fibreoptic and videolaryngoscope and patient cannot be ventilated using the LMA or facemask, a surgical airway is indicated. Hence, the difficult airway tray should always include a cricothyroidotomy kit.

a. Assessment of equipment: It is vital to check the functionality of all equipment to be used for the procedure and carefully arrange them. From the oxygen source, to the sunction machine to the laryngoscopes must be checked. Backup equipment like extra tubes of various sizes, different types of laryngoscopes and sizes of blades, different types and sizes of LMA must be available. Equipment failure is a known cause of critical airway incidents. In the case report by Fagbohun et al. [15], they experienced laryngoscope light source failure after an initial check of the said laryngoscope prior to commencing the procedure. However, they were able to seamlessly maneuver around the incident as there was a back up laryngoscope on their airway trolley.

b. Skills, Strategy and positioning: The airway managers must collaborate with other theater professionals to ensure a smooth and supportive inter personal relationship. The choice of airway management in patients should not only consider the anesthetists and patient but also consider the surgical access/field for the surgeons and adherence to established airway guidelines to facilitate effective airway management.

Air way managers have emphasized that proper positioning of the patient by maintaining jaw-lift, good neck positioning, use of continuous positive airway pressure, identifying a potential difficult airway before a procedure and outlining a care-plan based on the accepted difficult airway algorithm will reduce the risk of critical incidents during airway management especially in an environment where resources are scarce [16, 17].

It is appropriate to ensure adequate debriefing between all members of the peri-operative care team regarding the observed peculiarity of the patient, potential difficulties envisaged and possible resolution plans associated with the airway assessment.

4.3 Ethics and team members' roles/specification

Obtaining thorough and comprehensive informed consent from patients or their authorized legal care givers or decision makers is crucial before administering anesthesia and conducting an airway assessment. All team members should freely air their opinions and views to ensure patient has optimal care. All issues of concern should be discussed and resolved before the procedure begins. The role of each team member should be clearly specified during debriefing to ensure proper coordination [17, 18].

4.4 Preparation for extubation

The anaesthesiologist should consider the benefit of awake extubation to extubation while patient is still unconscious. The patient should be well ventilated to avoid critical incidents from hypoxia. Until the patient is fully recovered, the difficult airway tray should be maintained and within reach.

4.5 Follow up care

It is necessary that all difficult airway management experiences and how they were managed are properly documented. Detailed information should be given to the patient or responsible adult in the case of children or the incapacitated patient to guide future airway management. (Preferably as a document)The patient should also be evaluated for possible complications from the difficult airway management experienced [1, 17, 18].

5. Conclusion

Working in a resource scarce environment is challenging to the airway manager. It is important that these specialists working in these unique environments are constantly engaged in refresher courses to update their knowledge and skills on current standard practices and constant drills should be organized to put the knowledge acquired to test and use so that they do not forget the skills acquired. It is important to note that the best airway plan for the patient is dependent on the patient, the skill of the attending airway manager and the available equipment at the time of intervention and not just the availability of advanced airway equipment.

Author details

Omolola Fagbohun
Lagos State University Teaching Hospital/Lagos State College of Medicine, Ikeja, Lagos, Nigeria

*Address all correspondence to: lolafagbohun@yahoo.com

References

[1] American Society of Anesthesiologists Task Force on Management of the Difficult Airway. Practice guidelines for management of the difficult airway: an updated report by the American Society of Anesthesiologists Task Force on Management of the Difficult Airway. Anaesthesiology. 2003;**98**(5):1269-1277. Erratum in: Anesthesiology. 2004 Aug;101(2):565

[2] Cormack RS, Lehane J. Difficult tracheal intubation in obstetrics. Anaesthesia. 1984;**39**(11):1105-1111

[3] Cook TM, MacDougall-Davis SR. Complications and failure of airway management. British Journal of Anaesthesiology. 2012;**109**(1):68-85. DOI: 10.1093/bja/aes393

[4] Mallampati SR, Gatt SP, Gugino LD, Desai SP, Waraksa B, Freiberger D, et al. A clinical sign to predict difficult tracheal intubation: A prospective study. Canadian Anaesthetists' Society Journal. 1985;**32**(4):429-434

[5] Nørskov AK, Rosenstock CV, Wetterslev J, Astrup G, Afshari A, Lundstrøm LH. Diagnostic accuracy of anaesthesiologists' prediction of difficult airway management in daily clinical practice: a cohort study of 188 064 patients registered in the Danish Anaesthesia Database. Anaesthesia. 2015;**70**(3):272-281

[6] Bair AE, Caravelli R, Tyler K, Laurin EG. Feasibility of the preoperative Mallampati airway assessment in emergency department patients. The Journal of Emergency Medicine. 2010;**38**(5):677-680. DOI: 10.1016/j.jemermed.2008.12.019

[7] Kar S, Senapati LK, Samanta P, Satapathy GC. Predictive value of modified Mallampati Test and Upper Lip Bite Test Concerning Cormack and Lehane's Laryngoscopy Grading in the Anticipation of Difficult Intubation: A Cross-Sectional Study at a Tertiary Care Hospital, Bhubaneswar, India. Cureus. 2022;**14**(9):e28754

[8] Brain AI. The laryngeal mask – A new concept in airway management. British Journal of Anaesthesia. 1983;**55**:801-805

[9] Rachel M, Jarrod M, Darren B, Calvin A, Fred E. Crash a mnemonic for the physiological difficult airway. NRP. 2020;**2020**:1

[10] Rich JM. Recognition and management of the difficult airway with special emphasis on the intubating LMA-Fastrach/whistle technique: a brief review with case reports. Proceedings (Bayl Univ Med Cent). 2005;**18**(3):220-227

[11] Onyekwulu FA, Nwosu A. Emergency airway management with laryngeal mask airway. Nigerian Journal of Clinical Practice. 2011;**14**:95-97

[12] Chalam KS, Gupta J. Comparison of intubating laryngeal mask airway and fibreoptic bronchoscopy for endotracheal intubation in patients undergoing cervical discectomy. Journal of Anaesthesiology Clinical Pharmacology. 2016;**32**(4):515-518

[13] Yumul R, Elvir-Lazo OL, White PF, Sloninsky A, Kaplan M, Kariger R, et al. Comparison of three video laryngoscopy devices to direct laryngoscopy for intubating obese patients: A randomized controlled trial. Journal of Clinical Anesthesia. 2016;**31**:71-77

[14] Boehringer B, Choate M, Hurwitz S, Tilney PV, Judge T. Impact of

video laryngoscopy on advanced airway management by critical care transport paramedics and nurses using the CMAC pocket monitor. BioMed Research International. 2015;**2015**:821302

[15] Fagbohun O, Ibifuro D, Olugbusi S, Oresanwo T. Anaesthesia for reconstruction surgery post mandibulectomy in a patient with a predicted difficult airway: A case sreport. Integrated Journal of Medical Science. 2021;**8**:1-3

[16] American Society of Anesthesiologists Task Force on Management of the Difficult Airway. Practice guidelines for management of the difficult airway: An updated report by the American Society of Anesthesiologists Task Force on Management of the Difficult Airway. Anesthesiology. 2003;**98**:1269-1277

[17] Frerk C, Mitchell VS, McNarry AF, Mendonca C, Bhagrath R, Patel A, et al. Difficult Airway Society 2015 guidelines for management of unanticipated difficult intubation in adults. British Journal of Anaesthesia. 2015;**115**:827-848

[18] Nickson C. Airway assessment. In: LITFL – Life in the FastLane. Available from: https://litfl.com/airway-assessment/ [Accessed June 8, 2023]